ADVANCED FIRST AID
AND
EMERGENCY CARE

The American National Red Cross

AMERICAN RED CROSS

ADVANCED FIRST AID AND EMERGENCY CARE

Prepared by the American National
Red Cross for the Instruction
of Advanced First Aid Classes

First Edition 1973
With 353 Illustrations

Second Printing October 1973

DOUBLEDAY & COMPANY, INC.

Garden City, New York

ISBN: 0-385-05841-1 CLOTHBOUND
0-385-05902-7 PAPERBOUND

©1973 by
The American National Red Cross
All Rights Reserved
Illustrations © 1973 by
The American National Red Cross
Library of Congress Catalog Card No. 73-76727
Printed in the United States of America

PREFACE

Since 1910, the American National Red Cross has provided first aid instruction to the American public. The First Aid Program of the American National Red Cross, for which this book is a teaching text, stems from the Congressional charter provision that the organization shall devise and carry on measures for relieving and preventing suffering.

This textbook is designed for use by persons who are responsible for giving emergency care to the sick and injured. It provides the essential information for developing the functional first aid capabilities required by policemen, firemen, emergency squad and rescue squad members, and ambulance attendants. Emergency care instruction extending beyond the information given in this textbook should be provided by physicians and other specialized personnel.

To define current remedial procedures for this textbook, the Red Cross has asked the Division of Medical Sciences, National Academy of Sciences-National Research Council, to provide information for developing the content. The Division's assistance ensures the authoritative basis for the course content and provides a channel for extending the first aid recommendations of the medical profession to the American public.

The Red Cross expresses deep appreciation to members of the Ad Hoc Committee for Revision of the Red Cross First Aid Manual, under the chairmanship of Dr. Warren H. Cole, University of Illinois Medical Center, Chicago, Illinois, and to the staff of the Division of Medical Sciences. The Red Cross acknowledges, in particular, the contributions of Dr. Sam F. Seeley, Professional Associate, Division of Medical Sciences, for his technical guidance in developing this textbook prior to his retirement from the National Academy of Sciences. Thanks also are due to Dr. Virginia H. Blocker of Galveston, Texas, for her advice and assistance.

Appreciation for special assistance is also extended to the following Red Cross staff members: Thomas G. Parker, Albert S. Justus, Thomas D. Miller, and C. P. Dail, Jr.

John T. Goetz, director of the American National Red Cross First Aid Program, was responsible for the coordination of materials and the development of this textbook.

The book was illustrated by Angeline V. Culfogienis.

CONTENTS

1

INTRODUCTION TO FIRST AID

First aid is the immediate care given to a person who has been injured or suddenly taken ill. It includes self-help and home care if medical assistance is not available or is delayed. It also includes well-selected words of encouragement, evidence of willingness to help, and promotion of confidence by demonstration of competence.

The person giving first aid, the *first-aider*, deals with the whole situation, the injured person, and the injury or illness. He knows what not to do as well as what to do; he avoids errors that are frequently made by untrained persons through well-meant but misguided efforts. He knows, too, that his first aid knowledge and skill can mean the difference between life and death, between temporary and permanent disability, and between rapid recovery and long hospitalization.

NEED FOR FIRST AID TRAINING

Statistics show that accidents are the leading cause of death among persons from 1 year old to 38 years old; thereafter, accidents are one of the leading causes. The annual cost of medical attention, the loss of earning ability due to temporary or permanent impairment, the direct property damage, and the insurance costs amount to many billions of dollars each year, not to mention the toll in pain, suffering, disability, and personal tragedy.

Added to the grim accident statistics is the fact that the pattern of medical care has changed. Individuals today require, and should demand, the best possible care. Equipment for diagnosis and treatment, which is needed to provide such care, is usually at a hospital. Moreover, the growing population and expanding health needs have not been balanced by a proportional increase in numbers of doctors, nurses, and allied health workers. It is not enough to say, "Call the doctor"; a doctor may not be available to come to the scene of the emergency.

VALUE OF FIRST AID TRAINING

First aid training is of value in both preventing and treating sudden illness or accidental injury and in caring for large numbers of persons caught in a natural disaster.

Self-Help

If you, as a first-aider, are prepared to help others, you are better able to care for yourself in case of injury or sudden illness. Even if your own condition keeps you from caring for yourself, you can direct others in carrying out correct procedures to follow in your behalf.

Help for Others

Having studied first aid, you are prepared to give others some instruction in first aid, to promote among them a reasonable safety attitude, and to assist them wisely if they are stricken. There is always an obligation on a humanitarian basis to assist the stricken and the helpless. There is no greater satisfaction than that resulting from relieving suffering or saving a life.

Preparation for Disaster

First aid training is of particular importance in case of catastrophe, when medical and hospital services are limited or delayed. Catastrophe may take the form of a hurricane, a flood, an earthquake, a tornado, an explosion, or a fire. It may also take the form of a single accidental death or a life-threatening illness. Knowing what to do in an emergency helps to avoid the panic and disorganized behavior that are characteristic of unprepared persons at such times. Knowledge of first aid is a civic responsibility. It not only helps to save lives and prevent complications from injuries but also helps in setting up an orderly method of handling emergency problems according to their priority for treatment, so that the greatest possible good may be accomplished for the greatest number of people.

Safety Awareness

First aid training not only provides you with knowledge and skill to give life support and other emergency care but also helps you to develop safety awareness and habits that promote safety at home, at work, during recreation, and on the streets and highways. In the promotion of safety awareness, it is important to closely relate three terms: cause, effect, and prevention.

Cause

As various types of injury and illness are studied, initially only the more likely causes are identified, mainly because of the diversity of circumstances that are present in most accident situations. Aside from the more likely and obvious causative conditions, there are related human and mechanical factors to consider, as well as factors beyond the control of man.

A primary consideration in determining the root cause of an accident is human failure: an act of thoughtless, careless, or unwise behavior. Human failure may involve an act of doing something—or perhaps not doing something. It can create danger to oneself as well as to others. A person may wantonly disobey some regulation or law that has been established for safety. People often fail to heed warnings and follow directions. Instruction in the safe use of an object or in safe conduct may be inadequate; supervision during the learning process may be ignored. Human failure can also involve such mental or physical conditions as fatigue, inattention, impatience, and structural or functional handicaps of the body.

The possibility of mechanical malfunctions or structural failures as contributing causes of accidents also requires consideration. Faulty design or engineering may create a built-in hidden hazard. Manufacturing or construction procedures could lack the quality control necessary to ensure safe performance or use. The raw material may contain some inordinate defect.

When the in-depth study of an actual or hypothetical accident situation identifies all the causative factors, it becomes possible to determine <u>what</u> can be done to eliminate, control, or avoid the hazards.

Effect

The immediate effects of an injury or sudden illness consist of changes in the body's structure and functions. These effects are dealt with in the material on first aid care, particularly in discussions of signs and symptoms. However, long-range—possibly permanent— effects are also involved in many situations. Permanent disability can make it difficult for a person to enjoy a fully active and productive life. The economic and social structure of the family unit is frequently disrupted. In an accident, mental anguish brought on by knowing that one may have contributed to another's death or disability can linger on through a lifetime.

When analysis carefully considers both immediate and long-range or permanent effects of injury or sudden illness, it becomes obvious why every possible effort should be taken to eliminate, control, or avoid a situation that is hazardous to oneself or to others.

Prevention

A better understanding of the overall accident problem is developed if all the circumstances surrounding various types of accidents are carefully studied, including the broad range of first aid care that may be required. With such understanding, a person is likely to think and act more carefully, thoughtfully, and wisely. He tends to become more concerned for his own personal safety, as well as for that of others. He is likely to become genuinely interested in creating a safer environment on the highway, in the home, at work, in school, and at play. He will have a more responsible attitude toward accident prevention.

The causes of an accident indicate what accident-producing conditions and activities require attention. Accident effects indicate why such conditions and activities deserve concerted attention. Preventive measures should include a consideration of how these conditions and activities can be eliminated, controlled, or avoided.

GENERAL DIRECTIONS FOR FIRST AID

As a first-aider, you may encounter a variety of problem situations. Your decisions and actions will vary according to the circumstances that produced the accident or sudden illness, the number of persons involved, the immediate environment, and the availability of medical assistance, emergency dressings and equipment, and help from others. You will need to adapt what you have learned to the situation at hand or will need to improvise.

Sometimes, prompt action is needed to save a life. At other times, there is no need for haste. Efforts in the latter case will be directed toward preventing further injury, obtaining assistance, and reassuring the victim, who may be emotionally upset and apprehensive, as well as in pain.

First aid begins with action, which in itself has a calming effect. If there are multiple injuries or if several persons are hurt, priorities must be set. If you are the first-aider in charge you should enlist the help of bystanders to make telephone calls, to direct traffic, to keep others at a distance if necessary, to position safety flares in case of highway accidents, and so on. You should provide life support to victims with life-threatening injuries, attending first to those suffering from stoppage of breathing and then to those with severe hemorrhaging. You can then turn to those with less critical injuries.

Telephone or have someone else telephone the appropriate authorities regarding the accident. The police department or the highway patrol is a good first contact, but the circumstances surrounding the accident should be a guide as to whom to call. You should always have a list of emergency telephone numbers available. If the numbers are not readily available, ask the operator for assistance. Describe the problem, indicate what is being done, and ask for whatever help you think is needed, such as an ambulance, the fire department, the rescue squad, or utility company personnel. Give your name, the location of the accident, the number of persons involved, and the telephone number where you can be reached. *Do not hang up the receiver* until after the other party hangs up, because he may wish to clarify some information.

Urgent Care

In case of serious injury or sudden illness, and while help is being summoned, you must *immediately*—

- Determine the best way of rescue (for example, removal of an accident victim from water, from a fire, or from a garage or room containing carbon monoxide or smoke).
- Ensure that the victim has an open airway and give mouth-to-mouth or mouth-to-nose artificial respiration if it is necessary.
- Control severe bleeding.
- Give first aid for poisoning or ingestion of harmful chemicals.

Specific emergencies that require immediate first aid will be discussed in the appropriate chapters in the text.

Additional First Aid Directions

Unless it is necessary for safety to move a victim at once, keep him in the position best suited to his condition or injuries. Do not let him get up or walk around. Protect him from aggravation of existing injuries. If blankets or covers are available, keep him warm enough to overcome or avoid chilling. If he is exposed to cold or dampness, place blankets or additional clothing over and under him.

If haste is not imperative, or after immediate problems are under control, survey the situation and try to find out exactly what happened. The direction and extent of the examination should be determined by the kind of accident or sudden illness and the needs of the situation. *Have a reason for what you do.* Information may be obtained from the victim or from persons who were present and saw the accident or the onset of illness. If the victim is unconscious and has no sign of external injury, try to obtain identification either from papers carried in the victim's billfold or purse or from bystanders, so that relatives may be notified. (It is advisable to have a witness when you are looking for identification.)

Many people with chronic illness, such as heart disease, may carry medication with them, to be taken in the event of sudden illness; or they may have emergency medical identification, such as a card or bracelet, that gives a clue to their condition.

Examine the victim methodically. Loosen constricting clothing but do not pull on the victim's belt, in case spinal injuries are present. Remove or open clothing as necessary to examine the victim and give first aid (clothing may be cut away or ripped at the seams) but do not expose the victim unduly without protective cover. (Discretion must always be used in removing clothing.) Note the general appearance (including discoloration) of the victim's skin and other signs and symptoms that may give a clue to the injury or sudden illness. In the case of a victim with dark skin pigmentation, it may be difficult to interpret changes in skin color; look for changes in the color of the mucous membrane, which is the inner surface of the lips, mouth, and eyelids. Use all other available information concerning signs and symptoms, the history of the accident, and the like.

Check the victim's pulse; if you cannot feel it in the wrist, check for a pulse of the carotid artery at the side of his neck. Is the victim awake, stuporous, or unconscious? Does he respond to questions? Look at the expression of his eyes and the size of his pupils. Examine his trunk and limbs for open and closed wounds and for signs of fractures.

If the victim is unconscious, look for evidence of head injury. If he is conscious, look for paralysis of one side of his face or body. See whether he shows evidence of a recent convulsion. (He may have bitten his tongue, producing a laceration.) Check the front of the victim's neck to determine whether he is a laryngectomee. (Most laryngectomees carry a card or other identification stating that they cannot breathe through nose or mouth.) Do not inadvertently block the stoma of a laryngectomee when carrying out other first aid, because blockage could cause death from asphyxiation (see chapter 5).

If poisoning is suspected, check for stains or burns about the victim's mouth and a source of poisoning nearby, such as pills, medicine bottles, household chemicals, or pesticides.

Apply emergency dressings, bandages, and splints as necessary, if they are available.

Decide whether it is absolutely necessary to move the victim before help arrives.

After you determine the nature of the victim's injuries or illness, your plan of action will be affected by the kind of accident or sudden illness and the needs of the situation. Another major factor influencing this plan is the availability of human and material resources.

The first aid worker is not expected to explain the victim's probable condition to bystanders or to reporters. He *is* expected, however, to remain in charge until the victim can be placed in the care of qualified persons (for example, a physician, an ambulance crew, a rescue squad, or a police officer) *or* until the victim can take care of himself or can be placed in the care of relatives. Meanwhile, proper first aid measures should include standard specific techniques that have been taught and that, in view of the circumstances, appear to be necessary.

Above all, as a first aid worker, you should know the limits of your capabilities and must make every effort to avoid further injury to the victim in your attempt to provide the best possible emergency first aid care.

2

WOUNDS

DEFINITION

A wound is a break in the continuity of a tissue of the body, either internal or external. Wounds are classified as open or closed. An open wound is a break in the skin or in a mucous membrane. A closed wound involves underlying tissues without a break in the skin or a mucous membrane.

CAUSES

Wounds usually result from external physical forces. The most common causes of wounds are motor vehicle accidents, falls, and the mishandling of sharp objects, tools, machinery, and weapons.

EFFECTS

Any injury, unless it is very minor, may be harmful not only to the tissues directly involved but also to the functions of the entire body. Wounds that threaten life include those that produce cessation of breathing, severe bleeding, shock, or damage to the brain, heart, or other vital organ.

The local effects of an open or closed wound may include loss of blood, interference with blood supply, destruction of tissue, nerve injury, functional disturbances, and contamination with foreign material. These effects often involve nearby uninjured tissues. Even superficial wounds sometimes take a week or more to heal. The healing process includes absorption of blood and serum that have seeped into the area, repair of injured cells, replacement of dead cells with scar tissue, and recovery of the body from functional disturbances, if there were any.

The two most serious first aid problems caused by open wounds are a large, rapid loss of blood, which may result in shock, and contamination and infection of exposed body tissue.

TYPES AND CAUSES OF OPEN WOUNDS

Open wounds range from those that bleed severely but are relatively free from the danger of infection to those that bleed little but have greater potential for becoming infected. Often the victim has more than one type of wound.

Abrasions

An abrasion (Fig. 1) results from scraping (abrading) the skin and thereby damaging it. Bleeding in an abrasion is usually limited to oozing of blood from ruptured small veins and capillaries. However, there is a danger of contamination and infection, because dirt and bacteria may have been ground into the broken tissues.

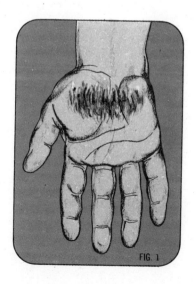

FIG. 1

Abrasions commonly result from falls or the handling of rough objects. Examples are skinned knees, rope burns (which are actually abrasions, not burns), and shallow multiple scratches.

Incisions

Incised wounds, or cuts (Fig. 2), in body tissues are commonly caused by knives, metal edges, broken glass, or other sharp objects. The degree of bleeding depends on the depth and extent of a cut. Deep cuts may involve blood vessels and may cause extensive bleeding. They may also damage muscles, tendons, and nerves.

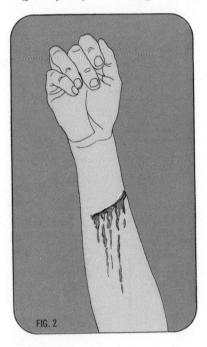

FIG. 2

Lacerations

Lacerations (Fig. 3) are jagged, irregular, or blunt breaks or tears

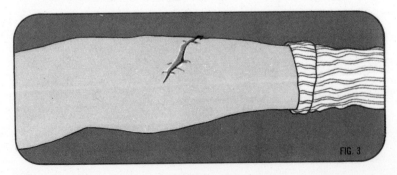

FIG. 3

in the soft tissues. Bleeding may be rapid and extensive. The destruction of tissue is greater in lacerations than in cuts. The deep contamination of wounds that result from accidents involving moving parts of machinery increases the chances of later infection.

Punctures

Puncture wounds (Fig. 4) are produced by bullets and pointed objects, such as pins, nails, and splinters. External bleeding is usually minor, but the puncturing object may penetrate deeply into the body and thus damage organs (as well as soft tissues) and cause severe internal bleeding. Because puncture wounds generally are not flushed out by external bleeding, they are more likely than some other wounds to become infected. Tetanus organisms and other harmful bacteria that grow rapidly in the absence of air and in the presence of warmth and moisture can be carried deep within body tissues by a penetrating object.

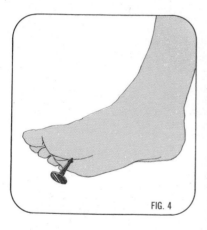

FIG. 4

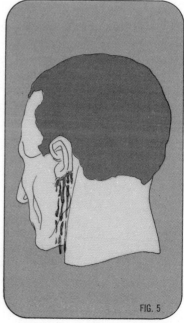

FIG. 5

Avulsions

Avulsion wounds (Fig. 5) involve the forcible separation or tearing of tissue from the victim's body. Avulsions are commonly caused by animal bites and accidents involving motor vehicles, heavy machinery, guns, and explosives. They are usually followed immediately by heavy bleeding. A detached finger, toe, nosetip, ear, or, in rare cases, whole limb may be successfully reattached to a victim's body by a surgeon if the severed part is sent with the victim to the hospital.

FIRST AID FOR OPEN WOUNDS

If the wound is in an inconspicuous location, is not deep, and gapes slightly, the first-aider may find that he need only hold the wound edges together and dress and bandage the injury. At times, however, it may be difficult for the first-aider to decide whether a wound needs medical care. He may ask himself, for example, whether it will need suturing by a physician. Identified below are a number of open-wound conditions that require medical treatment after emergency care has been provided:

- Blood spurting from a wound, even if controlled initially by first aid.
- Bleeding that persists despite all efforts to control it.
- An incised wound deeper than the outer layer of skin.
- Any laceration, deep puncture, or avulsion.
- Severed or crushed nerve, tendon, or muscle.
- Laceration of the face or other parts of the body where scar tissue would be noticeable after healing.
- Skin broken by a bite, human or animal.
- Heavy contamination of a wound by soil or organic fertilizer (manure).
- Foreign object embedded deep in the tissue.
- Foreign matter in a wound, not possible to remove by washing.
- Any other open-wound situation in which there is doubt about what to do.

Severe Bleeding

Loss of more than a quart of blood is a threat to a person's survival. Hemorrhage from the aorta (the largest blood vessel of the body) or from combined external and internal injuries (such as those in a gunshot wound) may be so rapid and extensive that the victim dies almost immediately. The loss of blood in some other kinds of wounds, such as the partial or complete severing of an arm or a leg, may not cause death as quickly, but large amounts of blood can be lost, and bleeding must be controlled. (For locations of the major arteries in the body, see Fig. 6.)

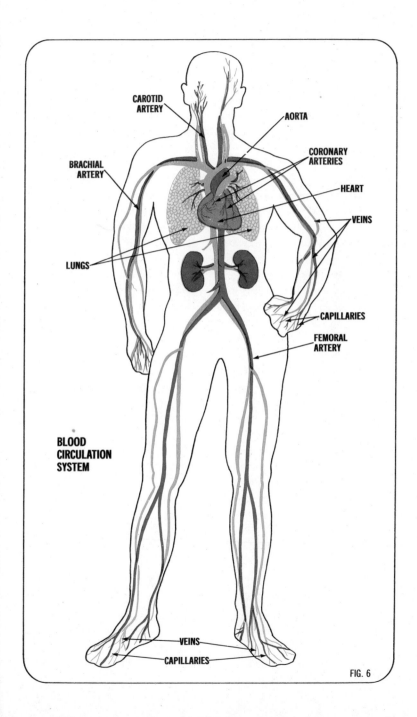

FIG. 6

The body of a victim who is bleeding severely can make some natural adjustments that help to slow down the blood loss. Even initial severe bleeding, such as the uncontrolled hemorrhage from a cut artery, may lessen or stop spontaneously. When a large blood vessel is completely severed, the normal elasticity of muscle layers in the vessel walls tends to make the cut ends retract. This retraction reduces the size of the opening through which blood can escape, and the flow of blood may slow down enough to permit clotting to begin. However, if a blood vessel is only partially cut, it will not retract to reduce the size of the opening, and bleeding will continue unless clotting occurs or the blood pressure decreases.

Blood pressure is another natural influence on bleeding. As the pressure drops, owing to the decreased volume of blood in the vessels, bleeding from the wound tends to slow down. A lowered pressure, however, is a grave sign, and death from severe shock is possible. In the case of some wounds that would be expected to bleed severely but are producing little or no evident loss of blood, the victim may already be in an advanced degree of shock. Such wounds must be watched carefully, because rapid bleeding may begin when measures to combat shock help to restore normal blood circulation.

First-aiders are urged to remember that a relatively small amount of bleeding, such as that from an open scalp wound, can make a victim look as if he were in a critical state, even when there is no danger of death due to bleeding. However, it is logical to assume that any loss of blood is harmful to the victim, inasmuch as it could interfere with the normal functioning of his circulatory system; and, because it is possible for a person to bleed to death in a very short period, blood loss of any extent should be stopped immediately.

Three distinct techniques are recommended to stop severe bleeding: direct pressure, elevation, and pressure on the supplying artery. A fourth technique, the use of a tourniquet, may be considered only when all other methods have failed to control severe bleeding. The four techniques are described below in order of preference.

Direct Pressure

Severe bleeding of an open wound can usually be controlled by pressing with the palm of one hand on a compress of cloth over the entire area of the wound (Fig. 7). A thick pad of sterile gauze is preferable, but any soft, clean cloth can be used in an emergency. Even unclean material can be used, but only if nothing better is immediately available.

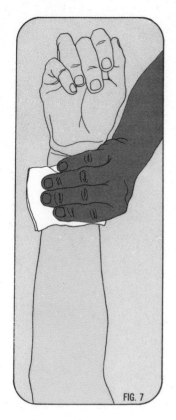

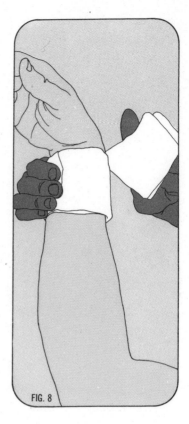

FIG. 7   FIG. 8

In an emergency, in the absence of compresses, the bare hand or fingers may be used, but only until a compress can be applied. Do not disturb blood clots that form in the cloth. If blood soaks through the entire compress, do not remove it; add more thick layers of cloth and continue direct hand pressure even more firmly (Fig. 8). The objective is to control the hemorrhage by compressing the bleeding vessels against something more solid, such as underlying bone or uninjured tissues.

The reason for applying hand pressure directly is to prevent loss of blood from the body without interfering with normal blood circulation. The first-aider is handicapped in carrying out other emergency care, and if such care is necessary, the compress should be secured in place by a pressure bandage. To apply the *pressure bandage*, place and keep the center of the bandage or strip of cloth directly over the pad on the wound; maintain a steady pull on the bandage to keep the pad firmly in place as you wrap the ends of it around the body part (Figs. 9 and 10). Tie the bandage with a knot directly over the pad (Fig. 11).

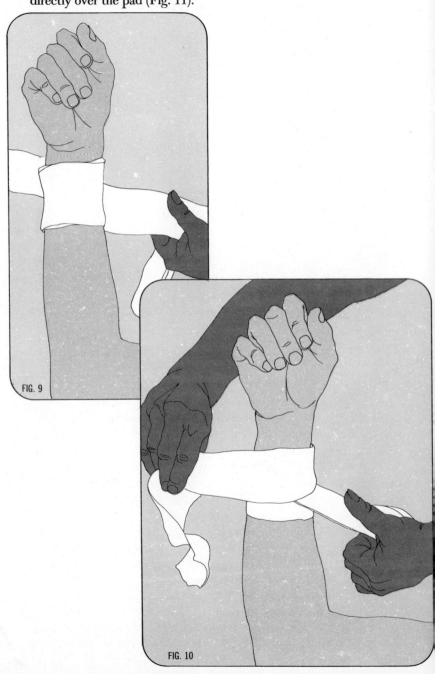

FIG. 9

FIG. 10

Elevation

Unless there is evidence of a fracture, a severely bleeding open
wound of the head, neck, arm, or leg should be elevated—that is,
raised above the level of the victim's heart (Fig. 12). Elevation uses
the force of gravity to help reduce the blood pressure in the injured
area and thus aids in slowing down the loss of blood through the
wound opening. However, direct pressure on a thick pad over the
wound must be continued.

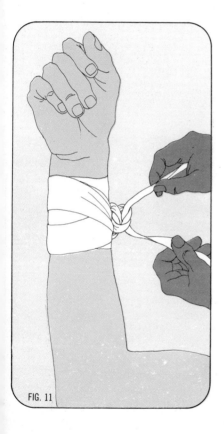

FIG. 11

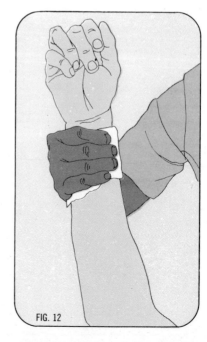

FIG. 12

Pressure on the Supplying Artery

If direct pressure and elevation do not stop severe bleeding from an open wound of the arm or leg, the pressure point technique may be required. This technique involves applying pressure at a specific point on the arm or leg to temporarily compress the main artery supplying blood to the affected limb. There is one recommended pressure point on each arm and leg (Fig. 13).

The use of a pressure point not only stops blood circulation to the injured limb but also stops circulation within the limb. Therefore, pressure points should not be used unless the technique is absolutely

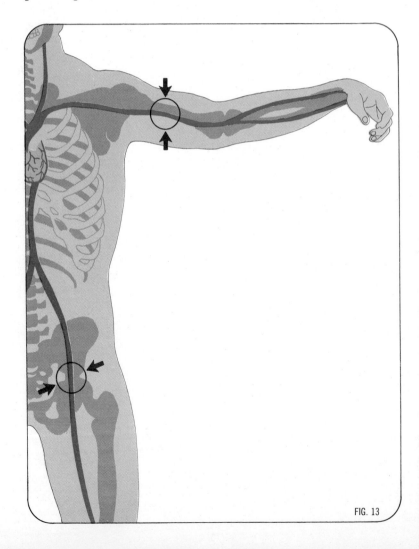

FIG. 13

necessary to help stop severe bleeding. If the use of a pressure point is necessary, do not substitute the technique for direct pressure and elevation but use it in addition to those techniques. You may need some help to apply all three control methods at the same time. As a rule, do not use a pressure point in conjunction with direct pressure and elevation any longer than is necessary to stop the bleeding, but be prepared to reapply pressure at the pressure point if bleeding recurs.

For a severely bleeding open arm wound, apply pressure over the brachial artery, forcing the artery against the arm bone. This pressure point is on the inside of the arm in the groove between the large muscle masses (biceps and triceps) about midway between the armpit and the elbow. To apply pressure on the brachial artery, grasp the middle of the victim's upper arm with your thumb on the outside of his arm and your other fingers on the inside. Press your other fingers toward your thumb to create an inward force from opposite sides of the arm. Use the flat inside surface of your fingers, not your fingertips. This pressure inward holds and closes the artery by compressing it against the arm bone (Figs. 14A and 14B).

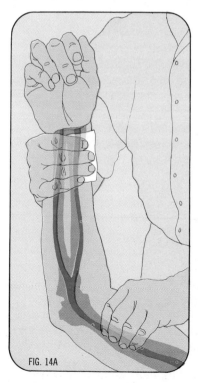

FIG. 14A

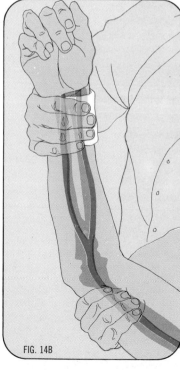

FIG. 14B

For severe bleeding from an open leg wound, apply pressure on the femoral artery, forcing it against the pelvic bone. This pressure point is on the front of the thigh just below the middle of the crease of the groin where the artery crosses over the pelvic bone on its way to the leg. To apply pressure on the femoral artery, quickly place the victim on his back and put the heel of your hand directly over the pressure point. Then lean forward over your straightened arm to apply pressure against the underlying bone. Apply pressure as needed to close the artery. Keep your arm straight to prevent arm tension and muscular strain (Fig. 15). If bleeding is not controlled, it may be necessary to compress directly over the artery with the flat of the fingertips and to apply additional pressure over the fingertips with the heel of the other hand.

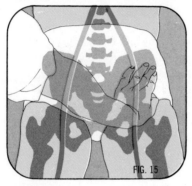

FIG. 15

Tourniquet

A tourniquet is a wide band of cloth or other material placed just above a wound to stop all flow of blood. Do not use a narrow band, rope, or wire. Application of a tourniquet can control severe bleeding from an open wound of the arm or leg *but is rarely needed and should not be used except in a critical emergency where direct pressure on the appropriate pressure point fails to stop bleeding.* The use of a tourniquet is dangerous. Properly applied, the tourniquet will stop all blood circulation to a limb beyond the point of application. But if it is left in place for an extended period, uninjured tissues may die from lack of blood and oxygen. Releasing the tourniquet tends to increase the danger of shock, and bleeding may resume. If a tourniquet is improperly applied (too loosely), it will not stop arterial blood flow *to* the affected limb, but will only slow or stop venous blood flow *from* the limb. The result is increased, instead of controlled, bleeding from the wound. *The decision to apply a tourniquet*

*is in reality a decision to risk sacrifice of a limb in order to save a life.
Once a tourniquet is applied, care by a physician is imperative.*

To apply a tourniquet, place it just above the wound. Do not
allow it to touch the wound edges. If the wound is in a joint area or
just below, place the tourniquet immediately above the joint.

- Wrap the tourniquet band twice tightly around the limb and tie
  an overhand knot (Fig. 16A).
- Place a short, strong stick—or similar article that will not break—
  on the overhand knot; tie two additional overhand knots on top of
  the stick (Fig. 16B).
- Twist the stick to tighten the tourniquet until bleeding stops (Fig.
  16C).
- Secure the stick in place with the loose ends of the tourniquet
  (Fig. 16D), a strip of cloth, or other improvised material (Fig.
  16E).

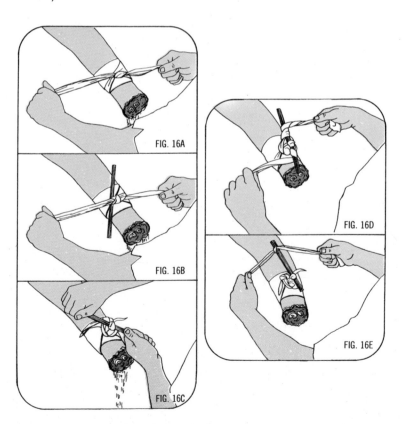

FIG. 16A

FIG. 16B

FIG. 16C

FIG. 16D

FIG. 16E

- Make a written note of the location of the tourniquet and the time it was applied and attach the note to the victim's clothing.
- Treat the victim for shock and give necessary first aid for other injuries.
- Do not cover a tourniquet.

Once the tourniquet has been applied, it *should not be loosened* except on the advice of a physician.

Prevention of Contamination and Infection

Open wounds are subject to contamination and infection. The danger of infection can be prevented or lessened by taking the appropriate first aid measures, depending on the severity of bleeding. Once a compress has been applied to control bleeding, whether bleeding has been severe or not, do not remove or disturb the cloth pressure pad initially placed on the wound. Do not attempt to cleanse the wound. The victim must have medical care, and cleansing the wound may cause resumption of bleeding.

A wound that is not bleeding severely and *that does not involve tissues deeper than the skin* should be cleansed thoroughly to remove contamination before it is dressed and bandaged, especially if medical attention will be delayed. Do not remove foreign materials from muscle or other deep tissues; such removal should be carried out only by a physician. To cleanse a wound that does not involve tissues deeper than the skin, wash your own hands thoroughly with ordinary hand soap or mild hand detergent. Wash in and around the victim's wound to remove bacteria and other foreign matter. Rinse the wound thoroughly by flushing with clean water, preferably running tap water. *Blot* the wound dry with a sterile gauze pad or clean cloth. Apply a dry sterile or clean dressing and bandage it firmly in place.

Caution the victim to see his physician promptly if evidence of infection appears (see page 40).

Removing Foreign Objects

In small open wounds, wood splinters and glass fragments often remain in the surface tissues or in tissues just beneath the surface. As a rule, such objects only irritate the victim; they do not usually incapacitate a person or cause systemic body infection. However, they can cause infection if they are not removed. Use tweezers sterilized over a flame or in boiling water to pull out any foreign matter from the surface tissues. Objects embedded just beneath the skin can be lifted out with the tip of a needle that has been sterilized in rubbing alcohol or in the heat of a flame. Foreign objects, regardless of size, that are embedded deeper in the tissues should be left for removal by a physician.

The fishhook is probably one of the more common types of foreign objects that may penetrate the skin. Often, only the point of the hook enters, not penetrating deeply enough to allow the barb to become effective; in this case, the hook can be removed easily by backing it out. If the fishhook goes deeper and the barb becomes embedded (Fig. 17), the wisest course is to have a physician remove it. If medical aid is not available, remove the hook by pushing it through (Fig. 18) until the barb protrudes. Using a cutting tool, cut

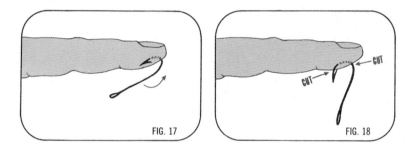

FIG. 17

FIG. 18

the hook either at the barb or at the shank and remove it. Cleanse the wound thoroughly and cover it with an adhesive compress. A physician should be consulted as soon as possible because of the possibility of infection, especially tetanus.

Some penetrating foreign objects, such as sticks and pieces of metal, may protrude loosely from the body or even be fixed, such as a stake in the ground or a wooden spike or metal rod of a fence on which the victim has become impaled. Under no circumstances should the victim be pulled loose from such an object. Obtain help at once, preferably from ambulance or rescue personnel, who are equipped to handle the problem. Support the victim and the object to prevent movements that could cause further damage. If the object is fixed or protrudes more than a few inches from the body, it should be held carefully to avoid further damage, cut off at a distance from the skin, and left in place. To prevent further injury during transport of the victim, immobilize the protruding end with massive dressings. The victim should then be taken to the hospital without delay.

Dressing the Wound

A dressing is a cover placed over a wound to protect it from additional injury and contamination and to assist in the control of bleeding. Bandaging a wound holds the dressing in place, assists in control of bleeding, offers support, and promotes restraint of movement. For detailed instruction on the application of dressings and bandages, see chapter 14.

INFECTION

The period of healing after an injury may be greatly prolonged by infection, which is the result of invasion and growth of bacteria within the tissues of the body. Bacteria are normally present in large numbers on the skin, in the nose, in the mouth, in the upper air passages, in the digestive tract, on hair, in hair follicles, in discharges from the body, in the air, and in soil. Serious infection may develop within hours or days after an injury, when bacteria get inside the tissues of the body through breaks in the skin or mucous membranes, even if the injury seems insignificant.

Careful cleansing of an open wound removes particles of dead tissue and foreign matter and reduces the number of bacteria, thereby helping to prevent infection. Bacteria tend to multiply rapidly in devitalized tissues; one reason is that white cells and other blood elements that ordinarily combat infection by destroying bacteria or by neutralizing bacterial products cannot reach dead tissues.

The threat of tetanus infection (lockjaw) must never be overlooked. A current immunization record will assist the physician in determining whether a tetanus injection or a tetanus toxoid booster injection should be given. Tetanus infection is so serious that a penetrating wound of any kind that involves tissues deeper than the skin should be seen by a physician as soon as possible.

Symptoms

Even if measures are taken to prevent contamination in a wound, infection may still develop. An infected wound can be recognized by the presence of any of the following symptoms:

- Swelling of the affected part.
- Redness of the affected part.
- A sensation of heat.
- Throbbing pain.

- Tenderness.
- Fever.
- Evidence of pus, either collected beneath the skin or draining from the wound.
- Swollen lymph glands ("kernels") in the groin (leg infection), in the armpit (arm infection), or in the neck (infection of the head).
- Red streaks leading from the wound—an indication that the infection is spreading through the lymphatic circulation channels.

Interim Emergency Care

Infected wounds require prompt medical care, but if a long delay is necessary before the victim can be treated by a physician, the following temporary steps should be taken:

- Immobilize the entire infected area and keep the victim lying down, preferably in bed, to reduce physical activity that would spread the infection.
- Elevate the affected body part, if possible. Elevation is especially important for infected wounds of the head, hands, legs, and feet.
- Apply heat to the area with hot water bottles, or put warm, moist towels or cloths over the wound dressing. Change the wet packs often enough to keep them warm and cover them with a dry towel wrapped in plastic, aluminum foil, or waxed paper to hold in the warmth and to protect bedclothing.
- Continue applying the warm packs for 30 minutes; then remove them and cover the wound with a sterile dressing for another 30 minutes. Apply the warm packs again. Repeat the whole process until medical care or advice can be obtained.
- If a physician is reached by telephone, be prepared to give him information about the victim's temperature and the general appearance of the wound.

Remember—the above directions are for interim care only; do not delay efforts to get medical care for the victim.

BITES

Injuries produced by animal or human bites may cause punctures, lacerations, or avulsions. Not only is care needed for open wounds but also consideration must be given to the dangers of infection, especially rabies.

Human

All human bites that break the skin may become seriously infected, because the mouth is heavily contaminated with bacteria. Cleanse the wound thoroughly, cover it, and seek medical attention.

Animal

The bite of any animal, whether it is a wild animal or a pet, may result in an open wound. Dog and cat bites are common. Although a dog bite is likely to cause more extensive tissue damage than a cat bite, the cat bite may be more dangerous, because a wider variety of bacteria is usually present in the mouth of a cat. Many wild animals, especially bats, raccoons, and rats, transmit rabies. Tetanus is an added danger in animal bites. Any animal bite carries a great risk of infection.

Rabies, or hydrophobia, is an infectious disease due to a virus. It can be transmitted through the infected saliva of a rabid animal to another animal or to a human being. The infection can be spread when the rabid animal's bite causes an open wound, even a scratch, or when the rabid animal licks an existing open wound on a human or a nonrabid animal.

The indications that an animal is rabid are variable and may be misleading. On the one hand, a rabid animal may drool, be irritable, be unusually active, or be clearly dangerous; on the other hand, it may be quiet, partially paralyzed, stuporous, or even affectionate. Every effort must be made to restrain any suspected rabid animal so that it can be kept under observation to see whether it develops the final stages of the disease. Do not kill such an animal unless it is absolutely necessary. If killing is necessary, take precautions not to damage the animal's head, which must be examined by public health authorities. Get help and advice from the police, a veterinarian, a physician, or local public health authorities as to how long a live animal that is thought to be rabid should be observed. Regulations vary from one community to another, but the average period is 15 days. If the animal cannot be caught for observation, arrange for immediate rabies immunization for any person it has bitten.

An animal in the final stages of rabies will develop some of the signs of the disease within 48 hours and will usually die within a few days after those signs appear. If the animal proves to be rabid, vaccine therapy must be given to build up body immunity in the victim in time to prevent the disease.

There is *no* known cure for rabies *once its final-stage symptoms develop.* After a person is bitten and the rabies virus is transmitted to him, the virus must go through an incubation period that may vary in duration. Any person who is bitten by an animal thought to be rabid should take no chances and should get medical care immediately. In the meantime, before a physician takes charge, thoroughly wash the wound with soap and water, flush it liberally, and apply a dressing. Movement of the arms and legs should be avoided until the victim has had medical care.

CLOSED WOUNDS

Most closed wounds are caused by external forces, such as falls and motor vehicle accidents. Many closed wounds are relatively small and involve soft tissues; the black eye is an example. Others, however, involve fractures of the limbs, spine, or skull and damage to vital organs (see page 44, Fig. 19) within the skull, chest, or abdomen. Massive injury to soft tissues—such as muscles, blood vessels, and nerves—can be very serious and can result in lasting disabilities.

Signs and Symptoms

Pain and tenderness are the most common symptoms of a closed wound. Usual signs are swelling and discoloration of soft tissues and deformity of limbs caused by fractures or dislocations. Suspect a closed wound with internal bleeding and possible rupture of a body organ whenever powerful force exerted on the body has produced severe shock or unconsciousness. Even if signs of injury are obvious, internal injury is probable when any of the following general symptoms are present:

- Cold, clammy, pale skin, very rapid but weak pulse, rapid breathing, and dizziness.
- Pain and tenderness in a part of the body in which injury is suspected, especially if deep pain continues but seems out of proportion to the outward signs of injury.
- Uncontrolled restlessness and excessive thirst.
- Vomiting or coughing up of blood or passage of blood in the urine or feces.

Emergency Care

Carefully examine the victim for fractures and other injuries to the head, neck, chest, abdomen, limbs, back, and spine. If an inter-

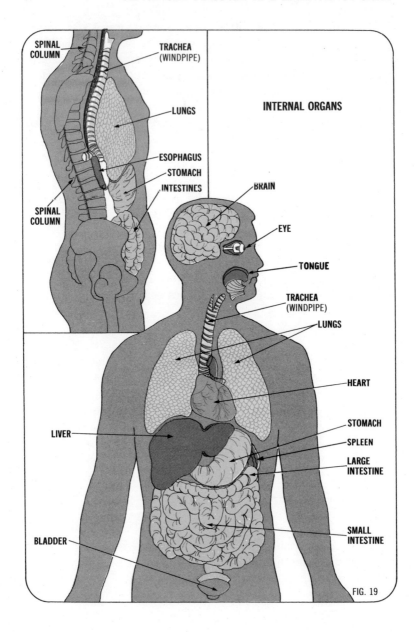

INTERNAL ORGANS

SPINAL COLUMN
TRACHEA (WINDPIPE)
LUNGS
ESOPHAGUS
STOMACH
INTESTINES
SPINAL COLUMN
BRAIN
EYE
TONGUE
TRACHEA (WINDPIPE)
LUNGS
HEART
LIVER
STOMACH
SPLEEN
LARGE INTESTINE
SMALL INTESTINE
BLADDER

FIG. 19

nal injury is suspected, get medical care for the victim as soon as possible. If a closed fracture is suspected, immobilize the affected area before moving the victim. Carefully transport him in a lying position and give special attention to preventing shock. Also, watch the victim's breathing and take measures to prevent either blockage of the airway or stoppage of breathing. Do not give fluids by mouth to a victim suspected of having internal injury, regardless of how much he complains of thirst.

When a relatively small closed wound occurs (such as a black eye), put cold applications on the injured area. The applications will help to reduce additional swelling and may slow down internal bleeding.

3

SPECIFIC INJURIES

EYE

Surface Irritation of the Eyeball

Eyes may be irritated by wind, dust, chemicals in the air, glare
from sun or lights, or contact lenses worn too long. Foreign objects
are often blown or rubbed into the eyes. Such objects are harmful,
not only because of the irritating effect but also because of the
danger of their scratching the surface or of becoming embedded.
Corneal ulcers may develop if the pupil area is involved. Surface
irritation of the eyeball can cause redness of the conjunctiva, sensitivity to light, a burning sensation, overproduction of tears, pain, and
headache.

In giving <u>first aid</u> when the surface of the eyeball is irritated, you
should observe the following precautions:

- Try to keep the victim from rubbing the eye. Rubbing may drive
  the foreign object into the tissues and make removal more difficult.
- Wash your hands thoroughly before examining the victim's eye.
- Do not attempt to remove a foreign object with a match, tooth-
  pick, or any other instrument.
- Refer the victim to a physician if something is embedded in the
  eyeball or if something is thought to be embedded but cannot be
  located.

To remove a foreign body from the surface of the eyeball or from
the inner surface of the eyelid—

- Pull down the lower lid and see, first, whether the object lies on
  the inner surface. If so, it may be lifted off gently with the corner
  of a clean handkerchief. Never use dry cotton around the eye.
- If the object has not been located, it may be lodged beneath the

upper lid. First, grasp the lashes of the upper lid gently between the thumb and forefinger while the victim looks down. Then pull the upper lid forward and down over the lower lid. Whatever is on the inside of the upper lid may be dislodged and swept away by tears. If the foreign body is not dislodged, depress the upper lid with a matchstick (Fig. 20A) or similar object placed horizontally on top of the cartilage, and evert the lid by pulling upward on the lashes against the matchstick (Fig. 20B). Lift off the foreign object with a corner of a clean handkerchief and replace the lid by pulling gently downward on the lashes.

- Flush the eye with water, using an eye dropper or small bulb syringe.
- If the object is still not removed, apply a dry, protective dressing and consult a physician.

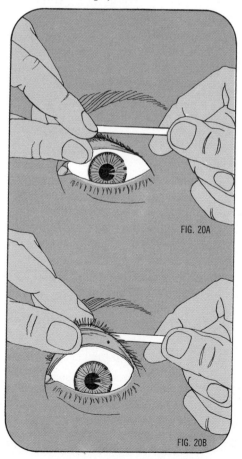

FIG. 20A

FIG. 20B

Injury of the Eyelid

Injury to the eyelid is much like other soft-tissue injuries, and the first aid treatment is similar: Stop bleeding by gently applying direct pressure. Cleanse the wound and apply a sterile or clean dressing, taped into place or held by a bandage that encircles the head. Seek medical care without delay. Treat bruises of the soft tissue above and below the eye that involve rupture of small blood vessels with immediate cold applications, to lessen bleeding and swelling.

Blunt Injury of the Eye

A blunt injury, or contusion, of the eye often occurs from a severe direct blow, as from a fist, in a vehicular accident, or in an explosion. The most common result is a black eye. In serious cases, the structure of the eye may be torn or ruptured; secondary damage may be produced by the effects of hemorrhage and later by infection. Vision may be lost. Because bleeding may begin even after several days, anyone experiencing a blunt injury of the eye should be seen by a physician, preferably an eye specialist, as soon as possible. In giving first aid, apply a dry sterile or clean dressing and have the victim lie down flat while he is transported to a place where he can receive medical aid.

Penetrating Injuries of the Eye

Penetrating injuries of the eye are extremely serious. If an object—such as a splinter of wood or steel, a BB shot, or a piece of glass—lacerates or penetrates the eyeball, the result may be some loss of vision or even blindness.

When giving first aid for such injuries—

- Make no attempt to remove the object or to wash the eye.
- Cover both eyes loosely with a sterile or clean dressing, secured with tape, or a bandage that encircles the victim's head but is loose enough to avoid pressure on the eyes. Coverage of *both* eyes is necessary to eliminate movement of the affected eye.
- Keep the victim quiet, preferably on his back. Transport him by stretcher.
- Call ahead to an eye specialist or take the victim to the nearest appropriate hospital emergency room. The sooner he receives medical care, the greater the chances of saving his sight.

HEAD

Scalp Injuries

Wounds of the scalp, even if small, tend to bleed profusely. A severe wound may be concealed by thick hair and may therefore be overlooked, especially if the victim has multiple injuries. Deep scalp wounds may be complicated by fragments of bone from skull fractures, or they may contain hair, glass, soil, or other foreign material. Do not attempt to cleanse such scalp wounds of contaminants. Cleansing can cause serious bleeding, and if the skull is fractured, can lead to contamination of the brain.

When giving <u>first aid</u>, treat severe hemorrhage of the scalp with the victim's head and shoulders raised, if possible, but do not bend the neck, since a fracture may be present. Place a sterile dressing snugly on the wound but be careful not to exert too much pressure against the underlying bone, because it may be fractured. When bleeding is under control, hold the dressing in place with a suitable temporary bandage to maintain the pressure.

Brain Injuries

Brain injury may be a factor not only in wounds of the scalp and open or closed fractures of the skull but also in illness, such as a stroke or a tumor.

In open skull fractures, there is often destruction of brain tissue, as well as laceration of the covering membranes. Such wounds are contaminated and present an enormous risk of infection. Associated injuries that result in lack of oxygen, owing to obstruction of the air passages or inadequate circulation of blood to the brain, can be extremely harmful. Lack of oxygen contributes to shock and may contribute to brain damage.

Clear or blood-tinged cerebrospinal fluid may drain from the nose or ears for several days after a skull fracture. No attempt should be made to pack the nose or ears or to stop the flow of fluid. The victim should be kept quiet, cautioned against blowing his nose, and placed under the care of a physician.

A temporary loss of consciousness almost always follows a severe blow on the head; this condition, in itself, does not necessarily indicate brain injury. A quick recovery of consciousness, even if there is confusion or temporary loss of memory, is a hopeful sign. If a person with a head injury loses consciousness later, his condition is probably serious because of progessive swelling of the brain or hemorrhage within the skull. Remember that bone cannot expand to accommodate swelling or accumulation of blood, as can the soft tissue of the body. If a person has suffered a blow to the head from any accident, major or minor, and a concussion or other brain injury is suspected, he should have medical attention and should be watched closely for from 24 to 48 hours.

Other manifestations of brain injury are—

- Partial or complete paralysis of muscles of the limbs on the side *opposite* that of the brain injury and of muscles of the face on the *same* side as the brain injury.
- Disturbance of speech. (The victim may know what he wants to say but may be unable to say it.)
- Convulsions, general or local (indicated by persistent twitching of muscles).
- Bleeding from the nose, ear canal, or mouth, which reflects possible head injury with a fracture.
- Pale or flushed face.
- Pulse that, although slow and full initially, becomes fast and weak.
- Headache, sometimes associated with dizziness.
- Vomiting.
- Pupils of the eyes unequal in size.
- Loss of bowel and bladder control.

When giving <u>first aid</u> for suspected brain injury—

- Keep the victim lying down and obtain medical assistance as quickly as possible.
- Call an ambulance equipped with oxygen.
- If there is no evidence of neck injury and the victim is unconscious, place a small pillow or a substitute (a rolled-up overcoat, a blanket, etc.) under his shoulders and head. *Do not* place the pillow only under the victim's head, because doing so might result in head flexion with consequent airway obstruction. Turn his head toward the side so that secretions may drool from the corner of his mouth. (Never position the victim so that his head is lower than the rest of his body.) Remove the pillow if artificial respiration is to be used.
- Give particular attention to ensuring an open airway. Administer artificial respiration when necessary.
- Control hemorrhage.
- If a dressing is needed for a scalp wound, lay a large dressing over the injury and apply a full head bandage.
- Loosen the victim's clothing around his neck and waist.
- Reassure the victim and handle him gently at all times.

- Check for associated injuries.
- Record the extent and duration of unconsciousness.
- Do not give the victim any fluids by mouth.
- Keep the victim warm but do not add extra heat. (Prevent chilling.)

FACE AND JAW (MAXILLOFACIAL AREA)

Victims of vehicular accidents or other types of violent injury often sustain soft-tissue wounds and fractures of the face and jaw, and there is always the possibility of a fracture of the neck. The principal immediate problems are obstruction of the air passage by blood, saliva, and other secretions, and swelling. In addition to pain and severe hemorrhage, a victim with fractures of the face or jaw will experience difficulty in speaking, in opening and closing his mouth, and in swallowing. The teeth may be irregular and deformed. When giving first aid—

- Ensure that the victim's air passages are open and remain open. Gently sweep your fingers through the victim's mouth to remove dentures, broken teeth, chewing gum, or other foreign objects.
- Wipe blood or other secretions out of the victim's mouth, as necessary, with a cloth or paper tissues; if a rubber bulb is available, use it for this purpose.
- Provide continuous support of the victim's head and jaw to prevent airway obstruction by the tongue.
- If the victim is conscious and neck injury is not suspected, prop him up so that he is leaning forward, to let blood and other secretions drain out spontaneously or when he coughs. (If the facial injuries are extensive, it should be assumed that the victim has a cervical spine fracture until X rays prove otherwise.)
- If the victim is unconscious, elevate his head and shoulders slightly (unless there is neck injury). Turn his head to the side so that blood and saliva may drain out. The victim may also be rolled on his side or abdomen for drainage.

NOTE. Jaw fractures and injuries that cause bleeding from the mouth or nose create special problems if artificial respiration must be given. Proper positioning and the gentle removal of foreign material or of blood clots may help to ensure an open airway, but the injuries may be such that it is difficult or impossible to administer mouth-to-mouth or mouth-to-nose artificial respiration. Under these conditions, the first-aider may have to resort to an alternative manual method of artificial respiration (see page 78).

- Treat the victim for shock, apply whatever protective dressings are necessary, and have someone call for an ambulance or medical assistance as quickly as possible. Persons with even small lacerations of the face need medical attention for suturing and protection from tetanus.

NECK

Collapse, swelling, and serious spasm of the larynx may result from pressure produced by blunt force over the throat. In such cases, remove any constriction. If necessary, use mouth-to-mouth or mouth-to-nose artificial respiration to revive the victim. Obtain immediate medical assistance in case an emergency tracheotomy (an opening into the trachea) is needed.

Lacerations or puncture wounds of the neck may involve the jugular veins, which are on the sides of the neck just beneath the skin, or the deeper major arteries and veins. Bleeding from neck wounds is dangerous and difficult to control. When giving first aid, control hemorrhage by direct pressure over the wound. Transport the victim to a hospital without delay and do not remove pressure until he is seen by a physician. If bleeding is not a problem, wounds may be covered by a dressing held in place with tape. Never apply a circular bandage around the neck.

Keep the victim's head and shoulders raised and his airway open.

MOUTH

Bleeding in the mouth can usually be controlled by direct pressure with a sterile or clean cloth. Lacerations of the skin and mucous membrane require suturing, as do large lacerations of the tongue and all gaping wounds. Small wounds of the mouth usually heal rapidly if there is thorough rinsing and proper attention to oral hygiene. Hemorrhage from a tooth socket after loss of a tooth can often be controlled by pressure on the area with a small pledget of gauze.

EAR

Cuts and lacerations of the ear are common. Any part of the ear torn off should be saved and sent with the victim to a medical facility. First aid consists of applying a dressing with light, even pressure and raising the victim's head. A tight dressing may cause additional injury to the ear.

Perforation (rupture) of the eardrum may result from a blast, a blow on the side of the head, a deep dive, a sudden change of pressure in an airplane, and middle ear disease. First aid consists of placing a small pledget of gauze or cotton loosely in the outer ear canal for protection until medical care is obtained. Do not allow the victim to hit himself on the side of the head to try to restore hearing; the blows may injure the delicate apparatus of the inner ear. Do not insert instruments or any kind of liquid into the ear canal.

A perforation of the eardrum associated with a skull fracture requires special attention. Cerebrospinal fluid may escape through the ear canal in some skull fractures. There is great danger of entrance of infection from the ear canal into the brain tissue. The canal *should not* be cleaned, and the flow of cerebrospinal fluid should not be stopped. Turn the victim gently onto the injured side (unless there is some specific reason not to), with his head and shoulders propped up on a small pillow or improvised pad, so that the fluid may drain away.

NOSE AND NOSEBLEED

Injury to the soft tissue of the nose may or may not include fractures. Avulsion of the tip of the nose is occasionally seen. Nosebleeds can result from injury or disease (such as high blood pressure, which can cause profuse, prolonged, and dangerous bleeding) or after a cold, a period of strenuous activity, or exposure to high altitudes. Nosebleeds are generally more annoying than serious. Walking, talking, laughing, blowing the nose, or otherwise disturbing clots may cause increase or resumption of bleeding. When giving first aid for nosebleed—

• Keep the victim quiet. Place him in a sitting position, leaning forward, whenever possible; if that is not possible, place him in a reclining position with his head and shoulders raised.
• Apply pressure directly at the site of bleeding by pressing the bleeding nostril toward the midline.
• Apply cold compresses to the victim's nose and face.
• If bleeding cannot be controlled by the above measures, insert a small, clean pad of gauze cloth (not absorbent cotton) into one or both nostrils and apply pressure externally with your thumb and

index finger. A free end of the pad must extend outside the nostril, so that the pad can be removed later.
• If bleeding continues, obtain medical assistance. A physician may be needed to pack the nasal cavity or cauterize the bleeding point.

Fracture of nasal bones often results in distortion unless the broken parts are properly repositioned. Deformity can cause difficulty in breathing. No first aid measures are needed, except, perhaps, a dressing. Nasal bone fractures, like all others, should have medical attention. If tissue has been avulsed, preserve it in a sterile dressing and send it to the hospital with the victim.

CHEST

Sucking Wounds

A sucking wound of the chest results from an open wound of the chest wall through which air may flow in and out with breathing (Fig. 21). Because the pressure inside the chest is normally lower

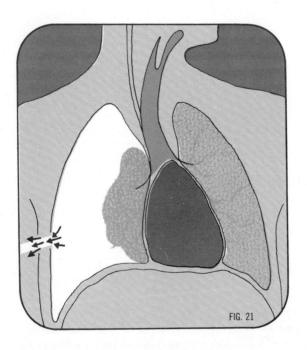

FIG. 21

than that outside, air is sucked in during inhalation, and the lung collapses and fails to function. Air in the chest cavity also compresses the unaffected lung, producing a serious emergency that requires prompt treatment. In giving first aid, close the wound opening with a large pad of sterile gauze or cloth (as clean as possible) or plastic or metal foil, applied with firm pressure and held in place with tape, a belt, or a bandage. Then place the victim on the affected side, if possible. Be careful not to apply the bandage so tightly that it restricts breathing. If necessary, use the palm of your hand until a suitable bandage can be obtained. Give artificial respiration if required. Remember that the sound of air passage at the stoma of a laryngectomee may be mistaken as a sucking chest wound, and the air passage must not be obstructed (see page 76). If respiratory difficulty becomes more profound soon after applying the airtight dressing, it may be because air is trapped in the chest cavity. This condition can be relieved by quickly removing, then replacing, the airtight dressing.

Penetrating Wounds

Serious penetrating wounds of the heart or the large blood vessels of the chest should be suspected if there is a puncture wound of the left side of the chest or of the back over the heart area, especially if such a wound is accompanied by signs of shock, internal hemorrhage, distention of the veins of the neck and arms, or faint heart sounds accompanied by a slow or imperceptible pulse. When giving first aid, if the wounding object or instrument is still in place, leave it undisturbed and immobilize it in place with dressings; removing it may result in fatal bleeding. Take the victim to the nearest hospital as quickly as possible and alert the staff in advance as to the nature of the emergency. Apply and secure a dressing firmly in place (with tape, if possible). Handle the victim gently and elevate his head and shoulders. Give artificial respiration if necessary.

Compression of Lung Tissue

A lung may be compressed by blood or other fluids or by air that has escaped into the chest cavity from the air passages through a tear in the surface of the lung. This emergency requires *immediate* medical attention, but until medical attention is available, any person with difficulty in breathing or with cyanosis (blue or ashen color of the skin, lips, or nail beds) should have first aid, as follows: Raise the victim's head and tilt it backward, with the neck arched. Clear the air passages and pull the victim's tongue forward, with the chin held up. Give artificial respiration if necessary.

Crushing Injuries

Crushing injuries commonly occur in vehicle accidents when a driver comes in contact with the steering wheel. These injuries of the chest restrict breathing because of the extreme pain. They are usually accompanied by rib fractures, which increase the pain and reduce expansion of the chest wall. When multiple rib fractures occur on both sides of the chest, the chest wall between the breaks will collapse, rather than expand, each time the victim attempts to inhale, which markedly reduces the volume of air exchange. This condition is known as a "flail chest."

First aid measures include placing the victim in a comfortable position. If fractures are on one side, it may be helpful to place the victim on the injured side, if possible. If the victim has a flail chest, splinting the fractured ribs may be helpful (see Fig. 105, page 172). If a bandage is required for an open wound, apply it carefully so as not to interfere with breathing. Elevation of the victim's head and shoulders may reduce his difficulty in breathing.

ABDOMEN

Wounds of the abdomen are dangerous because of the risk of damage to the internal organs. If a wound extends deep into the abdomen, in giving first aid, it is important to place the victim at rest, control bleeding, and give treatment for shock. The victim should lie on his back with a pillow or a pad under his knees to help relax the abdominal muscles. In open wounds of the abdomen, a first-aider should *not* try to replace protruding intestines or other abdominal organs (because of the danger of infection) but should cover them with a sterile dressing, a clean towel, or plastic or metal foil. Dampen the dressing if there is delay in obtaining medical assistance, using sterile or cool boiled water, if available. Hold the dressing in place with a firm bandage but do not make it tight enough to cause constriction. Do not give fluids or solid foods, because surgery will be necessary.

Occasionally, a person will have combined injuries of the chest and abdomen, and his breathing may be impaired by compression of the base of the lungs from below or from the chest injuries. If breathing difficulty develops, keep the victim's head and shoulders elevated with a pillow, a folded coat, or other improvised material.

Summon medical help as rapidly as possible and take extreme care to see that the victim is transported gently.

BACK

Open wounds of the back are usually caused by stabbing instruments, such as knives and ice picks, and by bullets or other missiles, as in industrial explosions. Closed wounds of the back commonly result from falls, traffic accidents, and injuries associated with sports, such as diving, skiing, and football. Fractures, dislocations, strains, sprains, and related conditions are discussed in chapter 13.

In any accident involving the back, injury to the spinal cord should be suspected. Such an injury may result in paralysis below the level of the wound, usually in association with fracture of the backbone (vertebrae). Very often, however, the cord is not as badly injured by the accident as by careless handling of the victim afterward *or* by bending the back during transportation.

If the victim of a back injury requires artificial respiration, it should begin in the position in which he is lying. If a person has been injured in the water, do not bend his head forward and do not place him in a jackknife position but float him to shore carefully and take him from the water only when a rigid support has been placed under his back (see chapter 6, page 87). Preferably, the victim should not be moved until an ambulance arrives with a special stretcher and trained personnel.

The kidney may be injured by blunt force applied to the back or by a penetrating object. The most common sign of kidney injury is a combination of severe pain in the side with muscle spasm, shock, internal hemorrhage, or blood in the urine. Handle the victim gently and seek medical aid as soon as possible.

GENITAL ORGANS

Injuries to the genital organs may result from kicks, blows, "straddle" accidents, accidents involving machinery, and, occasionally, blows from sharp instruments. The urethra or the bladder may be damaged, with leakage of urine and blood into the surrounding area. Such injuries are accompanied by great pain, marked swelling, and considerable bleeding. If any tissue has been torn loose, it should be saved for possible use in skin grafting of the injury. First aid for severe bleeding may require control by pressure with the hand or a pad of cloth. Other first aid treatment includes bed rest, application of cold packs, protective and supportive dressings for open wounds, and treatment for shock, if appropriate.

HANDS

The most important first aid for a hand injury is elevation of the hand above the level of the heart to reduce further swelling of the tissues. If the wound is extensive, do not try to cleanse it. Apply pressure over a sterile or clean pad to control bleeding. Place a roll of bandage, cloth, fluffed-up gauze squares, or other material into the victim's palm and curve his fingers around it. Separate the fingers by gauze or cloth dressing material and cover the entire hand with a sterile towel, clean cloth, or unused plastic bag. Elevate the hand in a sling or on pillows during transportation of the victim to obtain medical care.

Self-care for blood and water blisters should not be attempted if the blister fluid lies deep in the palm of the hand.

LEGS AND FEET

Serious wounds of the legs and feet are obviously disabling, but the importance of small wounds of the lower legs and feet is often overlooked. In older people, small wounds may take a long time to heal, because of poor circulation, and should receive medical attention. In giving first aid if medical treatment is delayed, cover wounds of the legs and feet and wrap the wounds with a supportive bandage, if available. Elevate the injured limb with pillows or a rolled-up coat.

Do not allow the victim with a leg or foot wound to walk. Make sure that bandages applied to hold dressings in place do not constrict. Remove the shoes and hose and examine the color of the victim's toes from time to time. If they become blue or swollen, loosen the bandages but do not remove dressings.

Blisters caused by friction from shoes or boots appear on the heels, toes, and tops of the feet. If all pressure can be relieved until the fluid is absorbed, it is best to leave blisters unbroken. Otherwise, in giving first aid, wash the entire area with soap and water; then make a small hole at the base of the blister with a needle that has been sterilized in a match flame or by being soaked in rubbing alcohol. Drain fluid and apply a sterile dressing to protect the area from further irritation. If the blister is already broken, treat it like an open wound and watch for signs of infection.

4

SHOCK

DEFINITION

Shock is a condition resulting from a depressed state of many vital body functions. It can threaten life even though the injuries or conditions that caused the depression may not otherwise be fatal. The vital functions are depressed when there is a loss of blood volume, a reduced rate of blood flow, or an insufficient supply of oxygen. Injury-related shock, commonly referred to as traumatic shock, is decidedly different from electric shock, insulin shock, and special forms of shock discussed in other sections of this textbook.

The degree of shock is increased by abnormal changes in body temperature, by poor resistance of the victim to stress, by pain, by rough handling, and by delay in treatment.

CAUSES

Shock may be caused by severe injuries of all types—hemorrhage, loss of blood plasma in burns or muscle swelling, or loss of body fluids other than blood (as in prolonged vomiting and dysentery); by infection; by a heart attack or stroke; by perforation of a stomach ulcer; by rupture of a tubal pregnancy; by anaphylaxis; or by poisoning involving chemicals, gases, alcohol, or drugs. Shock also results from lack of oxygen caused by obstruction of air passages or injury to the respiratory system.

EARLY STAGES

In the early stages of shock, the body compensates for a decreased blood flow to the tissues by constricting the blood vessels in the skin, soft tissues, and skeletal muscles. Their constriction causes an emergency redistribution of blood flow to the heart, brain, and other vital organs and may lead to the following signs:

- Pale (or bluish) skin, cold to the touch and possibly moist and clammy. (In the care of victims with dark skin pigmentation, it may be necessary to rely primarily on the color of the mucous membranes on the inside of the mouth or under the eyelids or of the nail beds.)
- Weakness.
- Rapid pulse (usually over 100), often too faint to be felt at the wrist (Fig. 22A) but perceptible in the carotid artery at the side of the neck (Fig. 22B) or in the femoral artery at the groin (see Fig. 13, page 34).

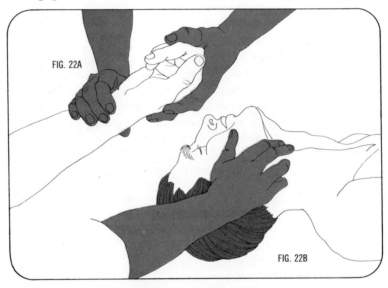

FIG. 22A

FIG. 22B

- Increased rate of breathing, possibly shallow, possibly deep and irregular. If there has been injury to the chest or abdomen, breathing will almost certainly be shallow, because of the pain involved in breathing deeply. A person in shock from hemorrhage may be restless and anxious (early signs of oxygen lack), thrashing about, and complaining of severe thirst, and he may vomit or retch from nausea.

LATE STAGES

If the victim's condition deteriorates, he may become apathetic and relatively unresponsive, because his brain is not receiving enough oxygen. His eyes will be sunken, with a vacant expression, and his pupils may be widely dilated (Fig. 23). Some of the blood

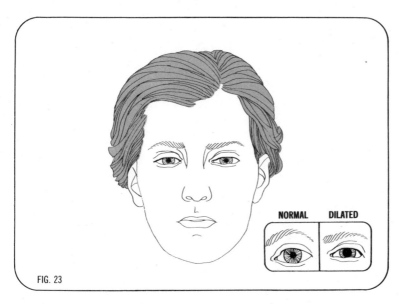

FIG. 23

vessels in the skin may be congested, producing a mottled appearance; this condition is a sign that the victim's blood pressure has fallen to a very low level. If untreated, the victim eventually loses consciousness, his body temperature falls, and he may die.

FIRST AID

The objectives of first aid care in shock are to improve circulation of the blood, to ensure an adequate supply of oxygen, and to maintain normal body temperature.

Give urgent first aid immediately to eliminate causes of shock, such as stoppage of breathing, hemorrhaging, and severe pain. Steps for preventing shock and for giving first aid for shock are as follows: Keep the victim lying down; cover him only enough to prevent loss of body heat; and obtain medical help. The victim's position must be based on his injuries. Generally, the most satisfactory position for the injured person will be lying down, to improve his blood circulation. If injuries of the neck or lower spine are suspected, *do not* move the victim until he is properly prepared for transportation, unless it is necessary to protect him from further injury or to provide urgent first aid care.

A victim who has severe wounds of the lower part of the face and jaw or who is unconscious should be placed on his side to allow drainage of fluids and to avoid blockage of the airway by vomitus and blood (Fig. 24). Extreme care must be taken to provide an open

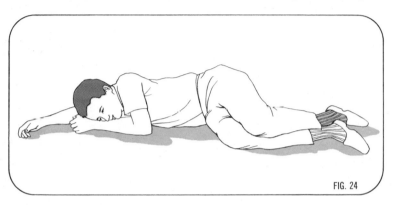

FIG. 24

airway and to prevent asphyxia. Place a victim who is having difficulty in breathing on his back, with his head and shoulders raised (Fig. 25). A person with a head injury may be kept flat or propped

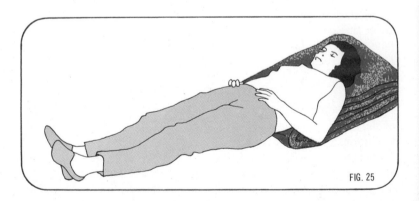

FIG. 25

up, but his head must not be lower than the rest of his body. A victim with severe brain injury may be unconscious, but unconsciousness is not in itself a cause of shock unless he also has associated fractures or major wounds. *If in doubt concerning the correct position on the basis of the injuries sustained, keep the victim lying flat.*

A victim in shock may improve with his feet (or the foot of the stretcher) raised from 8 to 12 inches (Fig. 26). This position helps to improve blood flow from the lower extremities. If in doubt as to whether the victim's feet should be raised, keep the victim flat. If he has increased difficulty in breathing or experiences additional pain after his feet are raised, lower them again.

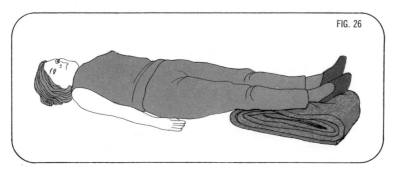

FIG. 26

Regulating Body Temperature

Keep the victim warm enough to overcome or avoid chilling. If he is exposed to cold or dampness, place blankets or additional clothing over and under him to prevent chilling (Fig. 27).

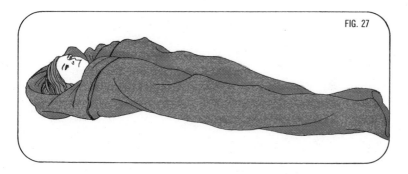

FIG. 27

Do not add extra heat, because raising the surface temperature of the body is harmful. Heat draws the diverted blood supply back to the skin from the more vital organs, thus robbing them of critically needed blood.

Administering Fluids

Although giving fluid by mouth has value in shock, fluids should *only* be given when medical help or trained ambulance personnel will not reach the scene for an hour or more. Other exceptions are when victims are unconscious, have convulsions, are vomiting, or are likely to vomit. (They may aspirate fluids into the lungs.) Do not give fluids to victims who are likely to require surgery or a general anesthetic or who appear to have abdominal injury. Oral fluids are harmful after injury to the brain, because additional fluids in the body may increase swelling of the brain. (A person with brain injury is likely to be unconscious or vomiting.) Fluids may be given by mouth *only* if medical care is delayed for an hour or more and none of the above contraindications exist.

Water—preferably water that contains salt and baking soda (1 level teaspoonful of salt and 1/2 level teaspoonful of baking soda to each quart of water) and that is neither hot nor cold—is recommended. Adults may be given about 4 ounces (1/2 glass) every 15 minutes; children, ages 1 to 12, 2 ounces; infants, 1 year or less, 1 ounce. Discontinue if nausea or vomiting occurs.

The preferred method is intravenous administration of fluids, a technique that provides intravascular volume restoration. However, this technique must be used only by individuals with specialized training and with authority.

5

RESPIRATORY EMERGENCIES
AND ARTIFICIAL RESPIRATION

DEFINITIONS

A *respiratory emergency* is one in which normal breathing stops or breathing is so reduced that oxygen intake is insufficient to support life.

Artificial respiration is a procedure for causing air to flow into and out of the lungs of a person when his natural breathing is inadequate or ceases.

CAUSES OF RESPIRATORY FAILURE

Anatomic obstruction is interference with breathing caused by the tongue's dropping back and obstructing the throat (one of the most common causes of respiratory emergency) or by swelling of tissues, which causes narrowing of the upper air passages. Constriction (narrowing) of the air passages may be caused by many conditions, such as acute asthma, croup, diphtheria, spasm of the larynx (as in allergic reactions that produce anaphylaxis), swelling after facial burns, swallowing of corrosive poisons, and direct injury caused by a blow (from a hand or a blunt instrument).

Mechanical obstruction is most commonly produced by partial or complete blockage of the air passage by a solid foreign object lodged in the pharynx or in any part of the airway but it may also result from the accumulation of fluids—such as mucus, blood, or saliva—in the back of the throat or from inhalation of vomitus.

Each year, nearly 2,000 deaths by asphyxia occur in the United States, because breathing is obstructed by liquids or solid objects, including food, caught in the larynx or esophagus or aspirated into the air passages. Sudden death may be caused by obstruction of the air passages directly or by pressure of a foreign body within the esophagus, which lies behind the trachea. Two-thirds of the deaths reported are in children under the age of 4.

Small children have a tendency to investigate objects by putting them into the mouth. Infants are often given articles such as candy, cookies, and toys by older brothers and sisters. Children cannot chew well until they have developed sufficient teeth (usually by about the age of 2), and grinding movements of the jaws are not effective until the child has grown the 4-year molars. Any inedible substance may be caught in the esophagus as a child attempts to swallow it, or it may be aspirated into the larynx accidentally, while he is laughing, crying, running, or jumping.

A foreign object that is accessible to your fingers should be removed if possible, but great care must be exercised in removing it, because either the pressure on the object or swallowing efforts may force the object more deeply into the throat (see page 76).

All small objects about the home are potentially dangerous for young children—nails, needles, coins, keys, marbles, glass and plastic articles, birthday-candle holders, beads, earrings, hairpins, paper clips, bottle caps, rubber bands, religious medals, buttons, weeds, grass, seeds (especially watermelon seeds), stems and pits of fruit, dried beans and dried kernels of corn used for play, fragments of shell and bone in food, and many more objects.

Mechanical obstruction of food and air passages in adults usually occurs when they swallow unchewed meat or food containing splinters of bone or shell—particularly when unexpected, as in chicken soup, salads, or sandwiches—or when they chew on nonedible objects as a nervous habit. Older persons with dentures are more likely to choke on food or bones, because normal sensation is diminished by the plates, and vision is likely to be impaired unless glasses are worn during eating. Eating without dentures is also hazardous.

Aspiration of solid objects into the lower air passages is not always obvious at first. (In some instances of choking on food, for example, a heart attack has been diagnosed on the basis of the victim's sudden collapse with marked chest pain, difficulty in breathing, and bluish discoloration of the face.) Foreign bodies are usually trapped by a spasm of the muscles at the level of the larynx. Coughing is a protective mechanism by which a foreign body is sometimes expelled from the larynx. A bean, peanut, or similar object drawn into the lungs causes either acute or chronic complications, but there might be no obvious symptoms for a long period.

A true life-threatening emergency exists when a person is choking and having difficulty in breathing. An inability to speak is a sure indication that the larynx is obstructed.

Breathing air depleted of oxygen or containing carbon monoxide or other toxic gases may cause asphyxia. Natural, slow oxidation processes sometimes remove the oxygen from the air in wells, cisterns, sewers, mines, and silos. If the air is not changed through ventilation, it will not support life, whether toxic gases are present or not. Plastic bags and other materials that may cause asphyxia when placed over the nose and mouth should be kept out of the reach of small children. Refrigerators and freezers with doors that cannot be opened from the inside are often the cause of accidents involving children and should never be abandoned unless the doors have been removed.

In addition to the dangers of asphyxia from carbon monoxide or from displacement of oxygen by natural oxidation processes or by other gases, there is often an explosion hazard. Combustible gases that accumulate in confined spaces—such as mines, cisterns, sewers, or rooms where natural or manufactured gas is free in the air—are explosive in some concentrations. Explosion may result if a flame is introduced, if static electricity is discharged, or if an electric switch, doorbell, telephone, or other electric device is used.

Additional causes of respiratory failure include—
- Electrocution.
- Drowning.
- Circulatory collapse (shock).
- Heart disease.
- External strangulation, as in hanging.
- Compression of the chest, caused, for example, by a mine cave-in.
- Disease or injury to the lungs. (Inadequate ventilation may be caused by an injury that collapses or compresses lung tissue, an injury that permits air to enter through a sucking wound of the chest wall, accumulation of blood in the chest cavity from hemorrhage, or an inflammatory disease of the lung, such as pneumonia.)
- Poisoning by drugs that depress respiration, such as morphine, opium, codeine, barbiturates, alcohol, and other narcotics.

THE BREATHING PROCESS

Contraction of the chest muscles and the diaphragm causes enlargement of the chest cavity. The diaphragm is a muscular partition that forms the floor of the chest cavity and separates the chest cavity from the abdomen. During the inhalation phase of breathing (inspiration), the chest muscles lift the ribs, expanding the chest. At the same time, the diaphragm, which is dome-shaped, contracts and descends toward the abdomen (Fig. 28). In this way, the chest cavity is increased in size, and atmospheric air flows in. When all the muscles relax, the ribs and diaphragm resume their former positions, the chest cavity becomes smaller, and air flows out (Fig. 29).

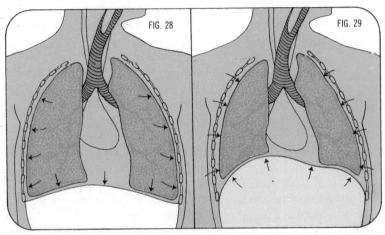

FIG. 28   FIG. 29

The average adult, at rest, breathes about from 12 to 18 times per minute; children breathe somewhat faster. Breathing rate varies greatly with exercise, excitement, and disease. Approximately 1 pint of air is inhaled with each breath by a resting adult, but not all this air actually enters the lung tissue. For artificial respiration to be effective, the volume of air that enters must exceed the amount that is already in the air passages and that is needed for normal respiration. Hence, air should be forced into the victim.

The body does not store oxygen but needs a continuous, fresh supply to carry on the life processes. Oxygen must be available to all body cells and is transported to them by the blood. The products of oxidation are heat, muscular energy, carbon dioxide, water, and some other chemicals. As air enters the body, it is 21 percent oxygen and 0.04 percent carbon dioxide. The remainder is largely nitrogen. The air that leaves the body is 16 percent oxygen and 4 percent carbon dioxide.

SIGNS AND SYMPTOMS OF RESPIRATORY EMERGENCIES

Regardless of the cause of a stoppage of breathing, the signs and symptoms will be characteristic of conditions in which breathing movements have stopped and lack of oxygen is present: the victim's tongue, lips, and fingernail beds become blue; there is loss of consciousness; the pupils become dilated.

ARTIFICIAL RESPIRATION

First aid for victims of carbon monoxide poisoning, overdosage of drugs, paralysis of the breathing muscles, or electric shock may include the application of prolonged artificial respiration. The objectives of artificial respiration are to maintain an open airway through the mouth and nose (or through the stoma) and to restore respiration by maintaining an alternating increase and decrease in the expansion of the chest.

Artificial respiration may be lifesaving if an accident or illness has caused cessation of breathing, and if the victim's body conditions otherwise permit life. In such a case, artificial respiration is necessary, because it will supply oxygen to the victim's body until his normal breathing process can resume.

Artificial respiration does not help if heart action has stopped completely, because then the blood no longer carries oxygen from the lungs to the body cells. Of all the body tissues, cells of the brain are the most sensitive to lack of oxygen. If breathing has stopped and the heart has not been beating for more than from 4 to 6 minutes, the brain is probably permanently damaged to the extent that, even if breathing resumes after this period, the victim might never recover consciousness.

Even though there may be doubt as to whether the heart is beating, artificial respiration should be attempted. However, giving cardiopulmonary resuscitation requires specialized training and should be carried out only by qualified persons (see page 80).

The mouth-to-mouth or mouth-to-nose technique of artificial respiration, in the absence of equipment, is the most practical method for emergency ventilation of a person of any age who has stopped breathing, regardless of why breathing has stopped. Extensive studies have indicated that mouth-to-mouth and mouth-to-nose resuscitation are unequivocally superior to any of the manual techniques. The mouth-to-mouth or mouth-to-nose technique provides more ventilation than other methods by using direct air pressure exerted by the rescuer to inflate the victim's lungs immediately. It also enables the rescuer to obtain more accurate information on the volume, pressure, and timing of efforts needed to inflate the victim's lungs than is afforded by other methods. Another advantage of this method of artificial respiration, aside from its effectiveness in ventilating the lungs, is that it may be given in the water, in a boat, underneath wreckage, and in other places where immediate resuscitation might be necessary.

The manual methods of artificial respiration are chiefly of historical interest because they are not as effective as the mouth-to-mouth or mouth-to-nose method. The manual methods do not provide as much ventilation as the mouth-to-mouth or mouth-to-nose method, and it is not possible to maintain an open airway at all times when the manual methods are used.

A manual method is *not* recommended except when the rescuer is unable to perform mouth-to-mouth or mouth-to-nose resuscitation for some reason, such as when massive facial injuries absolutely prevent the use of the mouth-to-mouth or mouth-to-nose method. If a manual method is justified, the preferred method would be the modified Silvester chest pressure-arm lift technique with a support beneath the shoulders to maintain backward tilt of the head. If a second rescuer is present, he should lift the lower jaw or maintain the head in the backward tilt position.

Mouth-to-Mouth (Mouth-to-Nose) Method

- Place the victim on his back.
- Wipe any obvious foreign matter from the mouth quickly (Fig. 30). Use your fingers, wrapped in a cloth if possible.

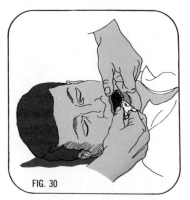

FIG. 30

- The tongue of the unconscious victim in the supine position may drop back and block the throat (Fig. 31A). To open the air passage, place one hand beneath the victim's neck and lift. Place the heel of the other hand on the victim's forehead and rotate or tilt his head backward into maximum extension—the head tilt method (Fig. 31B). Maintain the head in this position, since the position clears the airway by moving the tongue away from the back of the victim's throat. If additional airway opening is required, it can be achieved by thrusting the lower jaw into a jutting-out position—the jaw-thrust method (Fig. 31C).

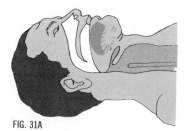

FIG. 31A

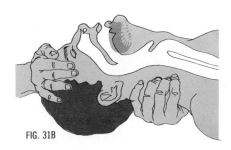

FIG. 31B

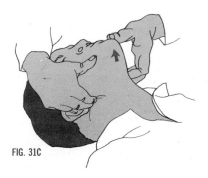

FIG. 31C

- For mouth-to-mouth ventilation, maintain the backward head-tilt position and, to prevent leakage of air, pinch the victim's nostrils shut with the thumb and index finger of your hand that is pressing on his forehead (Fig. 32A). This action prevents leakage of air when the lungs are inflated through the mouth. Another way to prevent leakage through the victim's nose is to press your cheek against his nose.
- Open your mouth widely, take a deep breath, seal your mouth tightly around the victim's mouth (Fig. 32B) and, with *your mouth*

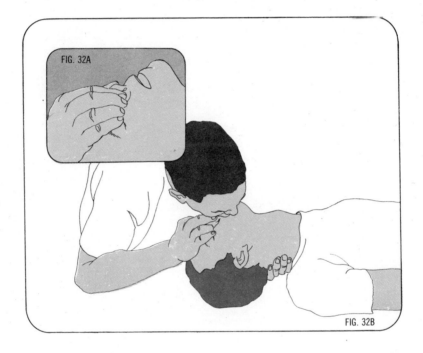

FIG. 32A

FIG. 32B

forming a wide-open circle, blow into the victim's mouth. Volume is important. You should start at a high rate and then provide at least one breath every 5 seconds for adults (or 12 per minute). If the victim's airway is clear, only moderate resistance to the blowing effort is felt.
- Watch the victim's chest. When you see it rise, stop blowing, raise your mouth, turn your head to the side, and listen for exhalation (Fig. 33). Watch the victim's chest wall to see that it falls.
- When the victim's exhalation is finished, repeat the blowing cycle.

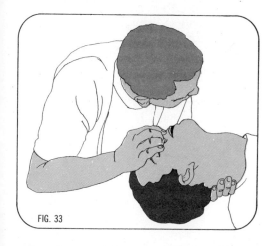

FIG. 33

- For the mouth-to-nose method, maintain the backward head-tilt position with the hand on the forehead. Use the other hand to close the mouth (Fig. 34A). Open your mouth widely, take a deep

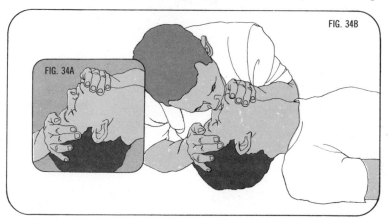

FIG. 34B

FIG. 34A

breath, seal your mouth tightly around the victim's nose, and blow into the victim's nose (Fig. 34B). On the exhalation phase, open the victim's mouth to allow air to escape (Fig. 35).

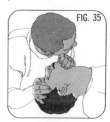

FIG. 35

- When administering mouth-to-mouth or mouth-to-nose ventilation to small children or infants, the first-aider should not make the backward head tilt as extensive as that for adults or large children.
- Both the mouth and nose of an infant or small child should be sealed by your mouth (Fig. 36). Blow into the mouth and nose every 3 seconds (or 20 breaths per minute) with less pressure and volume than for an adult or a large child, the amount determined by the size of the child. Small puffs of air will suffice for infants.

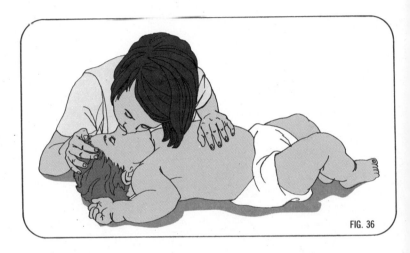

FIG. 36

The objective in positive pressure ventilation is to obtain a rise and fall of the chest. If the chest is not rising and falling during mouth-to-mouth or mouth-to-nose ventilation, something is wrong. The rescuer must quickly reassess the situation, again check for foreign matter, establish and maintain an open airway, and continue his blowing efforts.

- If you are not getting air exchange, recheck the position of the victim's head and jaw and investigate to see whether there is a foreign body in the back of the mouth obstructing the air passages.
- If the victim's stomach is bulging, air may have been blown into the stomach, particularly when the air passage is obstructed or the inflation pressure is excessive. Although inflation of the stomach is not dangerous, it may make lung ventilation more difficult and increase the likelihood of vomiting. If the stomach is bulging, turn

the victim's head to one side and be prepared to clear the mouth before pressing your hand briefly and firmly over the upper abdomen between the rib margin and the navel (Fig. 37). This procedure will force air out of the stomach but it may also cause regurgitation.

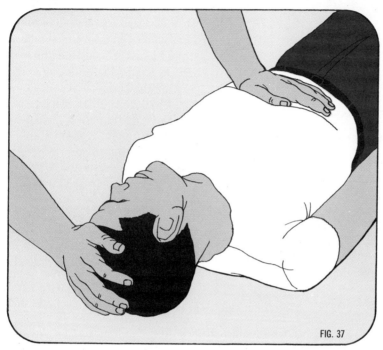

FIG. 37

- If a foreign body is completely preventing ventilation, turn the victim onto his side and use the heel of your hand to administer sharp blows between his shoulder blades over the spine (Fig. 38).

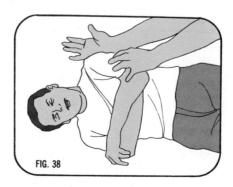

FIG. 38

The blows may jar the material free. A child may be turned upside down over one arm and given two or three sharp blows between his shoulder blades (Fig. 39). If still unable to ventilate, seek a foreign body that may be deep in the airway, and causing ob-

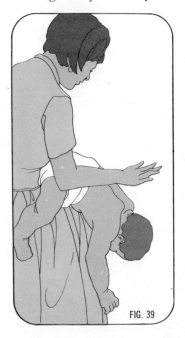

struction. Insert the index and middle fingers of one hand inside the victim's cheek and slide them deeply into the throat to the base of the tongue. Use a sweeping motion to carry them through the back of the throat and out along the inside of the other cheek to try to remove the foreign body. Clear his mouth again, reposition him, and repeat the mouth-to-mouth respiration.

FIG. 39

- Some persons who require artificial respiration never stop breathing completely but gasp irregularly. The gasping efforts actually assist in recovery but they should not encourage you to abandon mouth-to-mouth resuscitation until a normal pattern of respiration has been restored; however, *do not* attempt to blow in air whenever the victim is exhaling.
- *Do not* begin artificial respiration if it is definitely known that more than 30 minutes have elapsed from the time when breathing stopped. (The victim's pupils will be widely dilated and will not react to light; there will be no pulse in the neck vessels.) If the victim has rigor mortis, artificial ventilation need not be started.

Mouth-to-Stoma Method

In the United States there are about 25,000 persons whose larynxes have been completely or partially removed by surgery. The operation is called laryngectomy; those who have had the operation are called laryngectomees (Fig. 40). They breathe through an opening called a *stoma* in the windpipe (trachea) in the front of the neck and do not use the nose or mouth for breathing. There is no passage from the mouth and nose to the lungs. To speak, they use air in the esophagus. (Some are unable to talk at all.) Most laryngectomees

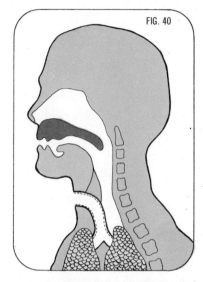

FIG. 40

carry a card or other identification stating that they cannot breathe through the nose or mouth.

If a person is wearing a breathing tube in his stoma, it may be clogged, causing breathing difficulties, especially in one who has undergone laryngectomy recently. It may be necessary for the first-aider to remove the tube by lifting it out with his fingers. The removal will open the airway and will not cause immediate danger. If the laryngectomee is conscious, he may want to clean the tube and replace it himself, and he should be permitted to do so. Otherwise, the first-aider should send the tube with the victim to a hospital for replacement in the stoma.

Because the stoma is low in the front of the neck and is the only means by which the laryngectomee can breathe, great care must be taken to avoid blocking it inadvertently. The sound of escaping air, especially in combination with secretions or blood flow after injury to this area, may lead one to conclude that the injury constitutes a sucking wound of the chest (see page 54) and therefore attempt to block the stoma with a pressure dressing. Blocking must be avoided, because it could lead to death from asphyxiation.

To give artificial respiration to a laryngectomee, do not breathe into his nose or mouth; you will only fill his stomach with air. Instead, use mouth-to-stoma respiration. Use the same general procedure as for mouth-to-mouth resuscitation but place your mouth firmly over the victim's stoma and blow at the same rate as for a person who breathes normally (Fig. 41), watching his chest for the

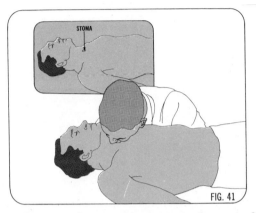

FIG. 41

inflow of air. This procedure is more sanitary than mouth-to-mouth breathing, because air coming from the stoma is cleaner than air coming from the mouth. Also, the contents of the laryngectomee's stomach cannot be vomited into the first-aider's mouth, because there is no connection between stomach and stoma. It is not necessary to tilt the head backward and to close off the victim's nose and mouth or to be concerned with his tongue or dentures. Keep the victim's head straight and avoid twisting his head; twisting might change the shape of the stoma or even close it.

The use of the Silvester method is justified only when the only first-aider available is also a laryngectomee. If the manual method is used, make sure to keep the victim's head straight.

Chest Pressure-Arm Lift Method (Silvester Method)

- If foreign matter is visible in the victim's mouth, wipe it out quickly with your fingers, preferably with a cloth wrapped around them.
- Place the victim in a face-up position. Maintain an open airway. An open airway can be maintained by placing something under the victim's shoulders to raise them several inches and allowing his head to drop backward (Fig. 42A). Turn the victim's head to the side.

- Kneel at the top of the victim's head, grasp the wrists, and cross them over the lower chest (Fig. 42B).

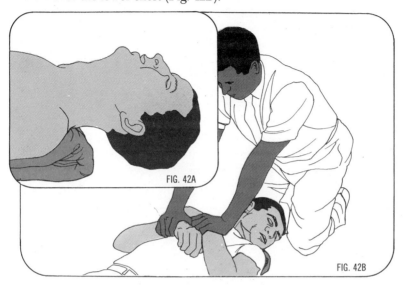

FIG. 42A

FIG. 42B

- Rock forward until your arms are approximately vertical and allow the weight of the upper part of your body to exert steady, even pressure downward (Fig. 43). This action will cause air to flow out of the victim's chest.

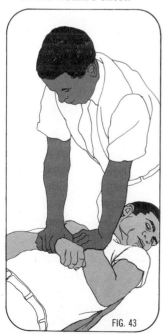

FIG. 43

- Immediately release this pressure by rocking back, pulling the victim's arms outward and upward over the victim's head and backward as far as possible (Fig. 44A). This procedure should cause air to flow in.
- Repeat this cycle about 12 times per minute, checking the victim's mouth often for obstruction.
- There is always danger of aspirating vomitus, blood, or blood clots. This hazard can be reduced by keeping the victim's head a little lower than his trunk. A helper should pull the victim's jaw forward and up and be alert to detect the presence of any stomach contents in the victim's mouth (Fig. 44B). The victim's mouth should be kept as clean as possible at all times. Remove any airway obstruction, as described in the technique for mouth-to-mouth breathing.

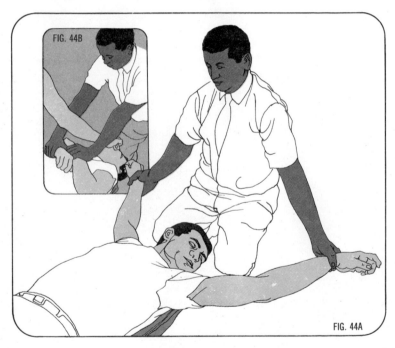

FIG. 44B

FIG. 44A

CARDIOPULMONARY RESUSCITATION

Cardiopulmonary resuscitation (CPR) is the combination of artificial respiration and manual artificial circulation that is recommended for use in cases of cardiac arrest. It requires special supplemental training in the recognition of cardiac arrest and in the performance of CPR. Instruction includes manikin practice in performing both individually and as part of a team. Periodic retraining is required unless rescuers have repeated experiences in the application of CPR.

Cardiopulmonary resuscitation involves the following steps:

A—Airway opening
B—Breathing restored
C—Circulation restored
D—Definitive therapy

External cardiac compression consists of the application of rhythmic pressure over the lower half of the sternum. This pressure compresses the heart and produces a pulsatile artificial circulation. External cardiac compression must always be accompanied by artificial ventilation.

Definitive therapy involves diagnosis, drugs, defibrillation (when indicated), and disposition. Definitive procedures are restricted to physicians or to members of allied health professions and authorized paramedical personnel under medical direction. The recommended basic techniques for performing the A and B steps are clearly defined in this text. The C and D steps are procedures requiring special supplemental training.

REMOVAL OF FOREIGN BODIES FROM THE THROAT

A foreign body, such as a piece of meat, that obstructs the respiratory passage above the level of the larynx provokes severe spasm of the muscles of the pharynx and the glottis. During this period of spasm, the foreign body is more tightly engaged and therefore more difficult to dislodge. If, during this period, the victim is coughing, choking, or otherwise trying to eliminate the foreign body, it is best not to interfere with his efforts and not to strike him on the back, and he should be encouraged to breathe slowly and deeply. If these efforts at expulsion cease and the victim becomes anoxic (oxygen deficient), semiconscious, or unconscious, he should be rolled onto his side (a child should be turned over the rescuer's forearm with the head down), and firm blows should be delivered over the spine between the shoulder blades. When the victim becomes anoxic, muscle spasm of the pharynx and glottis relaxes. It may then be possible to dislodge the foreign body with your finger, if it can be reached (see page 76), or by delivering blows over the spine.

Mouth-to-mouth or mouth-to-nose artificial respiration should be started promptly if the victim has difficulty in breathing, because air might bypass the obstruction sufficiently to maintain life or might force the aspirated material deeper into the airway, so that it will block one lung and allow ventilation of the other lung.

If the above measures fail, *sucking on the airway may be useful as a last resort.* Place the victim in a supine position with his mouth open; place a handkerchief or a light cloth over his mouth; put one of your hands on his stomach; and pinch his nostrils together with your other hand. Place your mouth on the victim's mouth and suck strongly on his airway, while at the same time you press downward on his stomach. The foreign object may be eliminated into the handkerchief covering the victim's mouth.

Even if relief is obtained after an episode of choking, the victim should get medical attention, because foreign material may remain, resulting in serious complications.

6

DROWNING, WATER ACCIDENTS, AND RESUSCITATION

DEFINITION

Drowning is a type of asphyxia related to either aspiration of fluids or obstruction of the airway caused by spasm of the larynx while in the water.

KINDS OF WATER ACCIDENTS

Drowning is a major cause of accidental death in the United States. It occurs in swimming, diving, boating, and other water activities, including ice skating, and usually in unsupervised water areas. Drownings can also occur in the home—in pools, bathtubs, and washtubs—and in water that is only a few inches deep.

CAUSES OF DROWNING

Drowning may occur under a number of circumstances. In some cases, people die in the water from a heart attack, a stroke, or overexertion. Fainting and epileptic attacks occur in water, just as they do on land; and loss of consciousness itself may result in accidental death. Occasionally, someone is struck by lightning while swimming or wading. Drowning may follow a head injury sustained in diving or in a collision with a log or other submerged object while swimming.

Cramps in the muscles of the hand, foot, calf, thigh, or abdominal wall may incapacitate a swimmer completely because of pain and fright, and he may double over with his head submerged and asphyxiate for lack of air. In cramping, muscles undergo marked spasm when they suddenly contract. Relief is usually obtained by stretching the involved muscles and applying firm pressure from the time the first twinges of pain are felt until the spasm is gone.

A drowning person may be seen either struggling in water and making ineffectual movements, floating face down on the surface of the water, or lying motionless underwater. Many persons sink very quickly as they lose buoyancy by swallowing water and by aspirating it into the lungs, where it replaces the tidal air (the volume of air normally inhaled and exhaled). The victim sinks beneath the surface and begins to lose consciousness from asphyxia. Effective motion ceases, and the specific gravity of the victim's body becomes greater than that of the water it displaces. Water pressure on the victim's chest wall increases as the victim descends, forcing air out of the lungs. The victim is unconscious but still may be revived if an attempt is made immediately.

Reflex Spasm of the Larynx

Asphyxia may occur from reflex spasm of the larynx, which closes the airway. This condition may occur immediately upon plunging into the water, especially if the water is cold, or as the result of pain, fear, or other conditions. Although the victim loses consciousness soon after he slips beneath the surface, his lungs may contain little or no water.

Submersion in Salt Water

If a person aspirates a large amount of sea water, the high concentration of salt will cause large amounts of fluid from his bloodstream to pass into and flood his lungs. Death may occur from shock, as a sudden fall in the blood pressure brings about circulatory collapse.

Submersion in Fresh Water

Fresh water sucked into a person's lungs enters his bloodstream and dilutes his blood. As the salt concentration of the blood lowers, red blood cells are destroyed. Water may be absorbed so rapidly that the victim's lungs are relatively dry. More commonly, tremendous swelling takes place, and frothy, pink-tinged fluid accumulates in his lungs as a result of ruptured red blood cells.

Adequate ventilation of the lungs after rescue may be impossible because of water blockage. Death may occur from either asphyxia or heart failure.

Hyperventilation

Drowning may result from excessive deep breathing or hyperventilation (overventilation) of the lungs before swimming underwater, diving, or testing how long the breath can be held underwater. When the carbon dioxide concentration of the blood is lowered by the forced exhaling of air during deep breathing, circulation of blood to the brain and the normal functioning of the brain may be greatly altered. Because of the mental confusion that can result, the underwater swimmer or diver may not recognize the usual warning signs that his oxygen supply is exhausted. These signs are a tight feeling in the chest, ringing in the ears, and acute air "hunger." The victim becomes confused, uncoordinated, and unconscious by stages; sometimes convulsions occur. The victim's mouth may open spontaneously as he makes strong efforts to inhale, and water is aspirated into the lungs. On land, a person who holds his breath to the point of unconsciousness ordinarily recovers completely without ill effect; submerged in water, he is asphyxiated and drowns.

FIRST AID

Immediately after rescue, begin artificial respiration, treat for shock, and transport the victim to a place where he can receive medical care. Water-accident victims who die usually do so within 10 minutes after the accident, from lack of air or from heart failure, not directly because of the presence of water in the lungs or the stomach. It is not possible to pour water out of the lungs, and no attempt should be made to do so.

Begin mouth-to-mouth respiration as quickly as possible in shallow water or while holding onto a boat or suitable buoyant aid. The rescuer must be alert to the possibility of an obstruction in the air passages and must act immediately if one occurs. Blow into the victim's mouth or nose more forcefully than in other types of emergencies affecting respiration, to force air through water in the air passages.

- After inflating the victim's lungs with 10 quick breaths, move to shore or pull the victim onto a suitable flotation device unless there is evidence of an injury to the spinal cord in the neck or back which requires a backboard or other rigid support.

- If the victim's stomach is bulging, turn him face down for a moment, place both hands under his abdomen, and lift his abdomen to assist in emptying his stomach (Fig. 45A); otherwise, air in

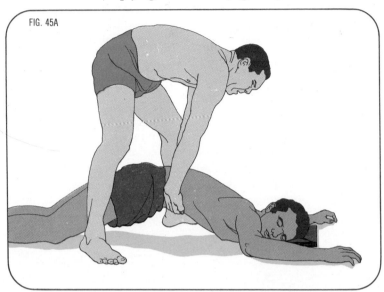

FIG. 45A

his stomach may interfere with both breathing and heart action. Another method is to leave the victim on his back, press on his stomach, and turn his head to the side (Fig. 45B).

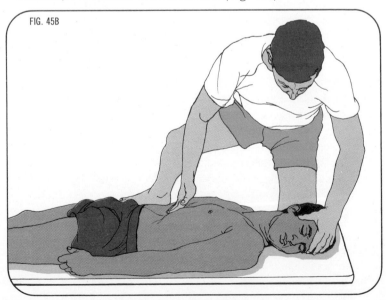

FIG. 45B

- Keep the victim from becoming chilled, apply artificial respiration continuously, and transport him to a place where he can receive medical care, as rapidly as possible.
- Do not allow a person who survives a near-drowning to walk.

Because delayed complications are common, the victim should be watched closely for several days, preferably in a hospital. Deaths that could have been prevented have occurred more than 48 hours after initial resuscitation, and such complications as pneumonia may develop.

NECK AND SPINE INJURIES IN WATER ACCIDENTS

Injuries resulting from water accidents require special first aid measures because of the frequent occurrence of cervical fractures, complicated by the possibility of drowning. Because cervical spine injuries are more likely to result in severing of the spinal cord than other vertebral fractures, protection against paralysis from spinal cord damage is imperative. Whenever possible, a trained assistant should be summoned and requested to bring a backboard, and the victim *should not* be removed from the water until the backboard arrives. If a backboard is not available, any rigid support may be adaptable, such as a wooden door, a surfboard, an aquaplane, a wooden plank, an ironing board, a picnic table bench, or any similar item that will not break or bend.

If the victim is floating face down, turn him over carefully with the least amount of movement, keeping his head and body aligned. Place one of your hands in the middle of the victim's back with your arm right over his head; place your other hand under the victim's upper arm, close to the shoulder, ready to turn him to the face-up position (Fig. 46). Rotate the victim by lifting his shoulder up and over with one hand while your other hand and arm support and maintain his head and body alignment (Figs. 47 and 48).

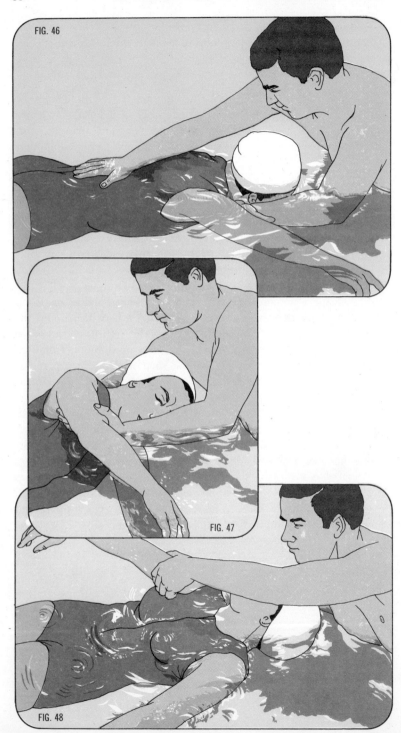

FIG. 46

FIG. 47

FIG. 48

The victim can be floated on his back in the water with minimal hand support. His head and neck should always be level with his back (Fig. 49), his airway must be kept open, and if mouth-to-mouth' resuscitation must be administered, use the jaw-thrust maneuver without head tilt. The backboard is placed under the victim by sliding it under the water and letting it float up (Fig. 50).

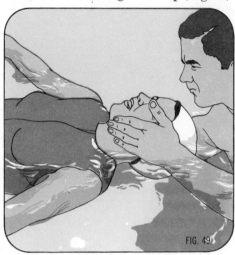

FIG. 49

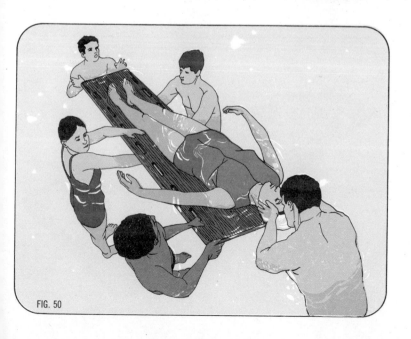

FIG. 50

Once it is in place, as an additional precaution to protect the victim from sliding or rolling, use any available material to secure his body to the rigid support (Figs. 51 and 52). Remove the victim from the water, keeping him as level as possible (Fig. 53). If rescuers are not trained and if there is insufficient help, it is best to keep the victim in the water until trained assistance is available.

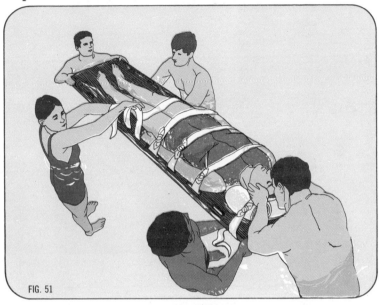

FIG. 51

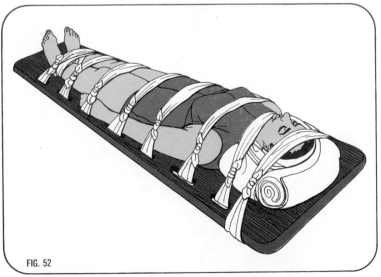

FIG. 52

However, there are some circumstances, such as excessive bleeding or water that is too cold, that may make it urgent to remove the victim from the water. Under such conditions, if no rigid support of any kind is available, constantly bear in mind the possibility of a cervical fracture and keep the victim's neck as nearly level with the back as possible by placing the heels of your palms at the back of his head and extending your fingers down onto his shoulders.

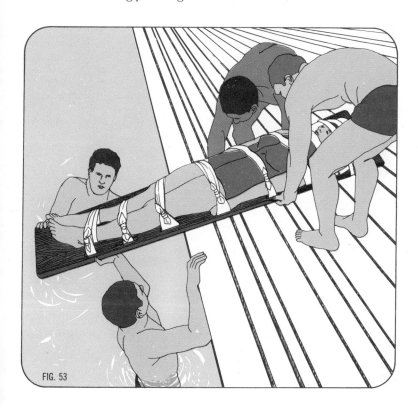

FIG. 53

WATER RESCUE

Most drownings occur within reach of safety; thus, rescue is often possible even if the first-aider is unable to swim. If a swimmer is in trouble near a dock or the side of a pool, lie down and extend your hand or foot to him, or hold out a towel, shirt, stick, fishing pole, float, deck chair, tree branch, or other object at hand and pull him to safety (Figs. 54A, 54B, and 54C). Use a line or ring buoy, if possible

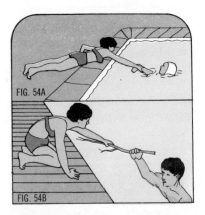

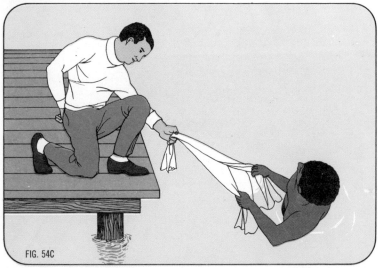

(Fig. 55). If the swimmer is too far from shore for these measures, wade into waist-deep water first with a suitable object to extend to him, push out a board to which he can cling while you go for help (Fig. 56A), or grasp his wrist and pull him to safety (Fig. 56B).

If a boat is available, row out to the victim and let him grasp the stern, or extend an oar and draw him around to the stern where he can hang on while you row to shore. If he is unable to hold onto the stern or the oar, pull him to the boat (Fig. 57) and, after checking for injuries, pull him into the boat.

If you are not trained in lifesaving, *do not* attempt a swimming rescue. Additional information can be found in the American National Red Cross textbook *Lifesaving and Water Safety*, which also includes a section on ice-accident prevention and rescue.

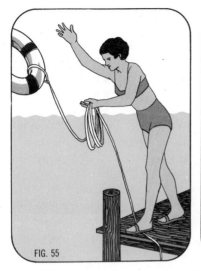

FIG. 55

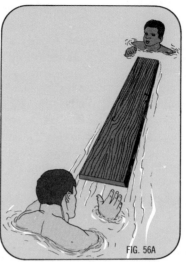

FIG. 56A

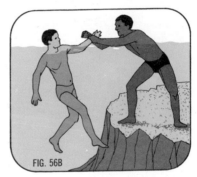

FIG. 56B

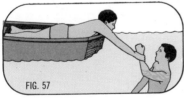

FIG. 57

ICE RESCUE

A useful device for ice rescue is a light ladder, from 14 to 18 feet long, with a light, strong line attached to the lowest rung. The ladder should be shoved out on the ice to the limit of its length, with the line serving as an extension. The rescuer may crawl out on the ladder to assist the victim (Fig. 58), if necessary. If the ice breaks under the ladder, the ladder will angle upward from the broken ice area and can be drawn to safety by other persons. Other usable rescue devices are buoys, ropes, sticks, poles, and even a human chain of rescuers lying prone on the ice.

Victims of skating accidents may require artificial respiration, which should be administered on the way to shelter, as well as warming and treatment for shock.

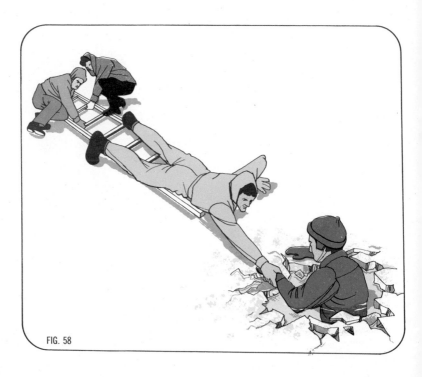

FIG. 58

7

POISONING

DEFINITION

A poison is any substance—solid, liquid, or gas—that tends to impair health or cause death when introduced into the body or onto the skin surface.

CAUSES

Serious poisoning may occur in a variety of ways; the most common is the ingestion, or swallowing, of a harmful substance. Volatile liquids—such as gasoline, kerosene, lighter fluids, turpentine, plastic glues, and paints—may enter the body by inhalation or swallowing or by a combination of the two. Some household chemicals, leaves, and berries are toxic when swallowed and may cause, on contact, an allergic reaction characterized by itching or a skin rash. Occasionally, poisoning results from an overdose of drugs, taken either accidentally or with suicidal intent.

Poisoning in children is the result of lack of supervision, negligence in storage or disposal of poisonous substances and curiosity combined with children's inability to read. The substances that most often cause poisoning in children are aspirin and other medications, cosmetics and hair preparations, gasoline, kerosene, and other petroleum products, paint and turpentine, and such common household chemicals as strong detergents, dry-cleaning agents, lye, bleaches, glue, washing soda, ammonia, acids, insecticides, and pesticides.

Many household products—such as strong detergents, bleaches, and cleaning solutions—may cause chemical burns of the skin and eyes. Pesticides, insecticides, and weed killers are particularly hazardous, because they can be absorbed through the skin, inhaled in sprays, or swallowed accidentally in large enough quantities to be fatal; and most of them have *no* known specific antidote. A number of these items have come onto the market only within recent years, and their names and actions are relatively unfamiliar to most persons. Many are chlorinated hydrocarbons and organic phosphates. They may cause sudden cessation of breathing, coma or convulsions, and rapid death. Every precaution should be taken in handling sprays—including their storage and mixing and the disposal of their containers—especially by farmers and others using these substances in large quantities.

Recent studies have shown many dangers from alcohol, in addition to chronic alcoholism. Alcohol in very small amounts affects physical and mental efficiency because it lowers the oxygen level in the bloodstream. Alcohol alone or in combination with carbon monoxide poisoning is often a factor in automobile accidents; alcohol combined with altitude is often responsible for small-plane accidents. The combination of alcoholic beverages with barbiturates or tranquilizers has been responsible for many deaths. (The odor of alcohol on the breath of an unconscious person does not mean, however, that he is intoxicated; some other serious medical problem may be responsible for the symptoms.)

INGESTED POISONS

Symptoms and Signs

The symptoms produced by swallowing poisons vary according to the type of poison, the length of time since ingestion, and the size of the person in relation to the amount ingested.

Food Poisoning

Distinguishing between food poisoning and other types of poisoning is sometimes difficult, because either may produce an unexplained sudden, severe illness accompanied by an explosive episode of nausea, vomiting, abdominal cramping pain, or diarrhea. Other substances, however, produce specific signs and symptoms that give a clue to the nature of the poison.

Corrosive Agents

Corrosive agents rapidly produce deep chemical burns of the victim's lips, mouth, and digestive passages when swallowed. These are strong acids and compounds with acidlike action—for example, rust removers, sulfuric acid, iodine, styptic pencil, some toilet bowl cleaners, and alkalies such as lye, washing soda, ammonia, bleaches, and strong detergents.

Petroleum Products

Kerosene, gasoline, and related petroleum products usually cause severe chemical pneumonia, as well as other toxic effects. These products may be identified by their characteristic odor.

Strychnine and Antihistamine Drugs

Many drugs may cause delayed convulsions, but strychnine and antihistamine drugs are the most familiar ones in which seizures may develop soon after ingestion.

Barbiturate Drugs, Opium-Derived Drugs, and Tranquilizers

Poisoning from barbiturate drugs, from paregoric or other opium-derived drugs (such as morphine and codeine), or from tranquilizers may be suspected if the victim is drowsy or in a coma and has slow, shallow breathing and slow pulse. After the victim has taken an overdose of morphine or similar drugs, his pupils contract to pinpoint size.

Belladonna or Atropine Poisoning

In belladonna or atropine poisoning, which may occur from some nonedible plants, as well as from medication, the victim's pupils are widely dilated, his pulse is rapid, and his skin is flushed, hot, and dry.

Aspirin

Signs of overdose of aspirin, which may be delayed for from 12 to 14 hours, include ringing in the ears, restlessness, rapid deep breathing, dryness of the skin, bleeding tendencies, and coma.

Poisonous Plants

Although poisonous plants rarely cause death, they may present a constant hazard to small children. The leaves, flowers, or fruits of many familiar flowers and shrubs—such as mountain laurel, rhododendron, oleander, some wild cherries, nightshade, and foxglove—

contain extremely toxic substances. Poisoning from mushrooms is also a potential risk to children and adults, unless one learns to distinguish between edible and nonedible types. Numerous plants that serve as sources of common medicines are poisonous in their natural state, because the active ingredients are highly concentrated and require dilution for safety. When eaten by grazing cows, the poisonous components of a few plants may be transmitted into milk and thus, indirectly, produce symptoms in persons who drink the milk.

First Aid

The objectives in first aid for poisoning by mouth are to dilute or neutralize the poison as quickly as possible, to induce vomiting (except when corrosive poisons are swallowed or when the victim is unconscious or having convulsions), to maintain respiration, to preserve vital functions, and to seek medical assistance without delay.

One person should begin to administer first aid immediately. If a second person is available, he should be directed to get advice by telephoning a physician, a hospital emergency room, or a poison control information center; to call for an ambulance; and to call the police if there are indications of suicide or homicide. If assistance is not available, give vital first aid immediately, and, as quickly as possible, obtain medical advice by telephone concerning antidotes and further action. The caller should give the following information:

- Age of the victim.
- Name of the poison and amount swallowed, if known—otherwise, the general nature of the poison.
- First aid being given.
- Information as to whether the victim has vomited.
- Your location and the time it will take to get to the doctor or the hospital and whether police escort will be necessary.

The label or container of the poison should be saved for identification. From what remains in the container, the amount taken may be estimated.

- If the victim is unconscious, keep his airway open; give him artificial respiration if it is warranted; transport him as quickly as possible to a place where he can receive medical help. Take along the poison container or a sample of vomitus if available.
- If the victim is having convulsions, do not give him any medication and do not induce vomiting. Arrange transportation as quickly as

possible. Do not attempt to restrain him but position him so that he will not injure himself by knocking against furniture or other objects. Loosen tight clothing at the victim's neck and waist. *Do not force a hard object or your finger between his teeth.* Watch for an obstruction of his airway. Give him artificial respiration if it is warranted. Do not give him anything to drink. *After the convulsion,* turn the victim on his side or face down, with his head turned to one side so that mucus will drain from his mouth.

If a noncorrosive poison—such as aspirin, snail bait, ant paste, or roach powder—has been swallowed—

• Dilute the poison by giving milk or water—three or four glasses for an adult; one or two glasses for a child.
• Induce vomiting. Insert the blunt end of a spoon or your finger into the back of the victim's mouth. If syrup of ipecac is available, it should be given in the dosage prescribed on the label. If you are unsuccessful in making the victim vomit after 5 *minutes,* take him immediately to a doctor or hospital. Do not wait for an ambulance if other transportation will take less time.
• When vomiting occurs, hold the victim face down with his head lower than his hips to prevent aspiration of vomitus into his lungs. An adult may lie across a bed with his head hanging over the side. Save a sample of the vomitus, as well as the poison container.
• Administer the specific antidote described on the label, in the case of poisoning by a commercial product, provided that the antidote is available; otherwise, have someone call a doctor, a poison control information center, or a hospital accident room for advice.
• Meanwhile, if you have either one on hand, give the victim activated medicinal charcoal or a commercial preparation called "the universal antidote," which contains medicinal charcoal as its most important ingredient. Give five or six heaping teaspoonfuls mixed with water in a thin paste—the same dose for children and adults. This preparation will absorb the poison. It is not harmful but it should be removed within a short time by flushing out the victim's stomach. Therefore, if it is not possible to get medical assistance promptly, induce vomiting again after 15 minutes. Do not give burned toast as a substitute for charcoal.
• Persons who have taken tranquilizers, barbiturates, paregoric, opium-containing drugs, or alcohol may be given coffee or strong tea as a stimulant *if they are conscious.*

If a corrosive poison, such as strong acid or alkali, has been swallowed—

- *Do not* induce vomiting. If the victim is conscious, give milk or water—two glasses for an adult, one glass for a child. Then egg white in water or cooking oil may also be given. If the victim has swallowed a strong alkali (for example, a drain cleaner, lye, washing soda, ammonia, bleach, or laundry or dishwasher detergent), water and vinegar or lemon juice may be given after the initial fluids. If a strong acid has been swallowed (for example, a toilet bowl cleaner), a weak alkali, such as milk of magnesia, may be given after the initial fluids.
- During transportation, treat the victim for shock; handle him gently; keep him from being chilled. Always keep his airway open. Anticipate vomiting and convulsions.

If a petroleum product or turpentine has been swallowed—

- *Do not* induce vomiting. Give the victim 4 ounces of mineral oil, if available; otherwise, give him milk or water—two glasses for an adult; one glass for a child.
- During transportation, treat the victim as described above.

INHALED POISONS

Sources

Poison gases, chiefly carbon monoxide and vapors from volatile liquids—such as gasoline, kerosene, lighter fluids, turpentine, plastic glues, and paints—result in 1,400 deaths a year in the United States. Because these statistics do not include suffocation in fires or deaths in transport vehicles in motion, it is obvious that the actual number is much greater. Of the reported group of deaths, almost half are from motor vehicle exhaust gas; one-fourth are due to incomplete combustion of gas in stoves used for cooking and heating. Possible sources of gas poisoning include—

- Carbon monoxide.
- Carbon dioxide (from wells, sewers, and industrial uses).
- Refrigeration gases in the home and in commercial ice-making and refrigerating plants—for example, ammonia and sulfur dioxide.
- Chlorine and related compounds (used in industry and in water purification).
- Solvents, such as carbon tetrachloride (used in fire extinguishers) and trichlorethylene.
- Anesthetic gases—for example, ether, chloroform, nitrous oxide, and cyclopropane.

- Fumes from sprays and liquid chemicals.
- Miscellaneous gases used in industry or produced as by-products of industry.
- Chemical-warfare agents—tear gas, nerve gases, blister gases, vomiting gases, lung irritants, hydrocyanic acid and other systemic poisons, screening smokes, and incendiary substances such as thermite and magnesium.

Carbon monoxide, the most common poisonous gas, is formed from incomplete combustion of fuels. It is particularly treacherous because it is completely odorless, and the victim may lose consciousness and be asphyxiated with no warning symptoms other than slight dizziness, weakness, and headache. Death may occur in a few minutes. Carbon monoxide combines very rapidly with the hemoglobin of the red blood cells, thus interfering with their oxygen-carrying capacity. The lips and skin of a victim of carbon monoxide poisoning are characteristically a cherry red.

The opportunities for carbon monoxide poisoning are prevalent. Particular precautions should be taken against inhalation of carbon monoxide in an automobile. Such inhalation may occur if there are defects in the vehicle's exhaust system, if the rear window is left down while driving in a station wagon, if a person drives at high altitudes with all the windows closed, and, above all, if a person runs the motor with the car standing still, either with the windows closed or in a garage or a confined space. Open fires and stoves, lanterns, charcoal grills for barbecue, and defective cooking equipment are other sources of carbon monoxide.

First Aid

- Remove the victim from the source of the poison, if possible; otherwise, call the fire department or a rescue squad.
- If the victim is in a closed room, garage, or other small space, take a breath and hold it before entering. Quickly turn off the motor of the automobile or the switch of the stove, if either one is the source of the poisonous gas, and pull the victim outside or to a place where there is fresh air.
- Have oxygen brought to the scene and seek medical assistance as rapidly as possible.
- Loosen the victim's tight clothing and clear his airway.
- If the victim has stopped breathing, give mouth-to-mouth artificial respiration.
- Treat the victim for contact poisons or chemical burns, if it is

warranted, by removing contaminated clothing and washing exposed areas of his skin.

CONTACT POISONS

Symptoms and Signs

Harsh chemicals and corrosive poisons can produce chemical skin burns that require immediate treatment.

Most reactions that follow contact with offending plants are allergic reactions and are characterized by itching, redness, rash, headache, and fever. Such reactions occur in susceptible persons from a wide variety of plant leaves, flowers, and berries, especially after they have been brushed against or crushed. The leaves of the stinging nettle, however, contain special hair cells that break off on contact and inject an irritating substance related to formic acid, found in ants and other stinging insects.

Some of the most common and most severe allergic reactions result from contact with plants of the poison ivy group, including poison oak and poison sumac. They produce a severe rash characterized by redness, blisters, swelling, intense burning, and itching. It has been estimated that 50 percent of the population is susceptible. The victim may develop a high fever and be acutely ill for several days, or even longer. Ordinarily, the attack begins within a few hours after exposure, but it may be delayed for from 24 to 48 hours. Sensitivity varies not only from one person to another but also in the same person from time to time.

The most distinctive feature of poison ivy and poison oak is their leaves, which are composed of three leaflets each. Both plants also have greenish-white flowers and berries that grow in clusters (Fig. 59).

First Aid

- Remove contaminated clothing. Drench and flush the affected skin immediately with large quantities of water or other available liquids as you remove clothing.
- Continue washing all contaminated skin with soap and water for at least 5 minutes.
- If poisoning is from a corrosive substance or a pesticide, send for an ambulance immediately.

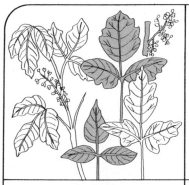

COMMON POISON IVY
(RHUS RADICANS)

• Grows as a small plant, a vine, and a shrub.

• Grows everywhere in the United States except California and parts of adjacent states. Eastern oak leaf poison ivy is one of its varieties.

• Leaves always consist of three glossy leaflets.

• Also known as three-leaf ivy, poison creeper, climbing sumac, poison oak, markweed, picry, and mercury.

WESTERN POISON OAK
(RHUS DIVERSILOBA)

• Grows in shrub and sometimes vine form.

• Grows in California and parts of adjacent states.

• Sometimes called poison ivy, or yeara.

• Leaves always consist of three leaflets.

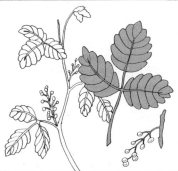

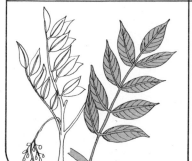

POISON SUMAC
(RHUS VERNIX)

• Grows as a woody shrub or small tree from 5 to 25 feet tall.

• Grows in most of eastern third of United States.

• Also known as swamp sumac, poison elder, poison ash, poison dogwood, and thunderwood.

FIG. 59

• Keep the victim's airway open. Give him artificial respiration if it is warranted. Do not leave him alone.

• Give the victim ample quantities of water or other liquids to drink *unless* he is having convulsions or is unconscious.

• In the case of poisoning by a pesticide or an unusual poison, save the label or a sample of vomitus.

In poisoning by poison ivy or poison oak—
* Remove contaminated clothing. Wash all exposed areas thoroughly with soap and water and apply rubbing alcohol.
* Apply calamine or other soothing skin lotion if the rash is mild.
* Seek medical help if a severe reaction occurs or if there is a known history of previous sensitivity.

POISONING BY MARINE LIFE

Current scientific explorations and the popularity of skin and scuba diving make it increasingly important to know of the dangers to be encountered in the sea. Contact with marine animals can produce puncture wounds (usually on the hands and feet), as well as toxic reactions. These reactions vary greatly, depending on individual sensitivity or resistance and on the virulence and amount of venom contacted.

Many species of fish are equipped with venom apparatus attached to dorsal or other spines—catfish, weever fish, scorpion fish (including zebra fish), toadfish, surgeonfish, and others. In many instances, little is known about the venom, and there are no known antidotes. First aid and treatment must, therefore, be related to the symptom.

Seasnakes, uncommon in waters bordering the United States, are of the cobra genus and inject an extremely potent venom that affects the nervous system. Treatment is the same as for other snakebites: immobilization with the affected area lower than the victim's heart, application of a constricting band (see Fig. 73, page 116), and medical assistance as soon as possible.

Ingestion of Poisonous Shellfish

Description, Signs, and Symptoms

Shellfish poisoning is related to bacterial contamination, allergic reactions, and a paralytic type of poisoning due to ingestion by clams and mussels of dinoflagellates, which are microscopic poisonous marine animals.

In paralytic poisoning, there is numbness of the victim's face and mouth (which spreads to other parts of the body), weakness, muscular paralysis, increased salivation, intense thirst, and difficulty in swallowing. The poison is concentrated in the dark meat, gills, digestive organs, and siphon of shellfish. The white meat is less harmful but should be washed thoroughly several times, and the

water in which it is cooked should be discarded. Shellfish poisoning
is unpredictable but is generally more common from March to
November than during the rest of the year.

Many varieties of shellfish should not be eaten. Learn the species
of marine life in your area that are known to be safe.

First Aid

First aid for ingested fish and shellfish poisons is the same as for
noncorrosive poisons (see page 99), except that persons who have
allergic reactions to scombroid fish (mackerel, for example) or
shellfish should seek medical advice regarding the administration of
an antihistamine.

Stings

Jellyfish and Portuguese Man-of-War

Jellyfish (Fig. 60A) and the Portuguese man-of-war (Fig. 60B) have
stinging cells—nematocysts (Fig. 60C)—on their tentacles that dis-
charge venom through threadlike tubes on contact, producing burning pain, a rash with minute hemorrhages in the skin, and, on

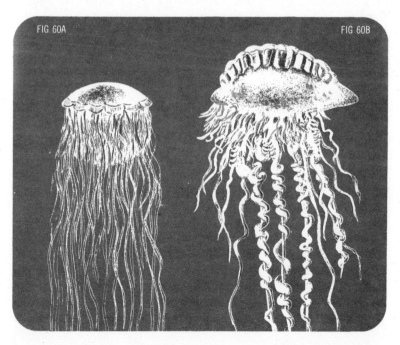

FIG 60A   FIG 60B

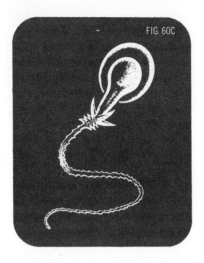

occasion, shock, muscular cramping, nausea and vomiting, and respiratory difficulty. Because tentacles may cling to the victim's skin, they should be gently removed with a towel, and the area should then be washed thoroughly with diluted ammonia or rubbing alcohol. A medicine for the relief of pain, such as aspirin, should be given. If symptoms are severe, seek medical aid.

Stinging Coral

Stinging coral—fire coral (Fig. 61A)—inject venom through stinging cells, producing multiple sharp cuts contaminated by particles of broken-off calcareous (calcium-containing) material. These cuts require thorough cleaning and prompt medical assistance. Anyone who works around coral should wear gloves, flippers or canvas shoes, and an outer garment for protection.

Cone Shell

The cone shell (Fig. 61B) is a type of mollusk related to the snail. It has a complicated apparatus for venom, which may be injected through a puncture wound. General symptoms include numbness and tingling about the victim's nose and mouth, and paralysis. Death from heart failure may occur.

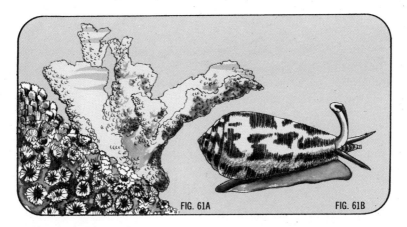

FIG. 61A   FIG. 61B

For first aid—

• Use a constricting band (see Fig. 73, page 116).
• Immediately soak the affected area in hot water for 30 minutes, or use hot compresses, because heat may help to inactivate the venom.
• If symptoms are severe, get medical aid.

Bloodworms

Bloodworms inflict a painful bite. After soaking wound in hot water, apply a constricting band (see Fig. 73, page 116).

Bristleworms

Bristleworms have stinging bristles that cause local inflammation and numbness.
For first aid—

• Remove the bristles with adhesive tape.
• Apply ammonia or alcohol to the affected area.

Sea Urchins

Sea urchins are equipped with sharp spines and multiple venom organs (pedicellariae) that contain a potent nerve poison.
For first aid—

• Treat the same as for cone shell poisoning.
• Seek medical assistance for severe symptoms and for removal of fragments of spines.

Stingrays

Stingrays (Fig. 62) inflict lacerations or punctures and inject toxic venom from glandular tissue that is an integral part of the caudal spine. General symptoms include shock, vomiting, diarrhea, and muscular paralysis. An occasional death is reported.

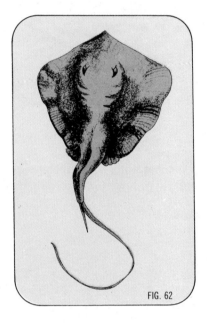

FIG. 62

For <u>first aid</u>—

- Soak the wounds in hot water.
- Control bleeding and apply a dressing.
- Obtain medical assistance for cleansing of the wound and for removal of fragments of the spine.

POISONING BY INSECTS

Kinds and Effects

Ants, Bees, Wasps, Hornets, and Yellow Jackets

Stings from ants, bees, wasps, hornets, and yellow jackets occasionally cause death. Deaths from the sting of such creatures is almost always due to acute allergic reactions or anaphylaxis in persons previously sensitized to insect proteins, rather than to the venom itself, except in the case of multiple stings of some ants.

Fleas, Mosquitoes, Lice, Gnats, and Chiggers

Stings or bites from fleas, mosquitoes, lice, gnats, chiggers, and other common insects produce local pain and irritation but are not likely to cause severe reactions. Some of these insects may transmit disease to man but are not harmful in themselves.

Ticks

Ticks (Fig. 63) are flat, usually brown, and about one-fourth of an inch long; they have eight legs. In some cases they can transmit germs of several diseases, including Rocky Mountain spotted fever, which occurs in the East as well as the West. They adhere tenaciously to the skin or scalp. There is some evidence that the longer an infected one remains attached, the greater is the chance that it will transmit the disease.

Black Widow and Brown Recluse Spiders

Spiders in the United States are generally harmless, with two notable exceptions: the black widow spider, Latrodectus mactans (Fig. 64); and the brown recluse, or violin spider, Loxosceles reclusa (Fig. 65). The black widow spider causes only slight local reaction but injects a nerve toxin that produces severe pain, profuse sweating, nausea, painful cramps of abdominal and other muscles, and difficulties in breathing and speaking.

Almost all victims recover, but an occasional death is reported. Reactions from bites of the brown recluse spider have been noted in increasing numbers in recent years, especially in the south central part of the United States. There have been a few deaths in children. The venom from this spider produces a severe local reaction that forms an open ulcer within from 1 to 2 weeks. Meanwhile, destruction of red cells and other blood changes take place. The victim may develop chills, fever, joint pains, nausea and vomiting, and even a generalized rash within from 24 to 48 hours.

Tarantulas

Tarantula (Fig. 66) bites ordinarily do not produce generalized reactions but may be responsible for severe local wounds and can be fatal. A number of tarantula bites are seen each year, particularly in persons who handle bananas and other fruit shipped from South and Central America.

Scorpions

Scorpions (Fig. 67) inject venom through a stinger in the tail. A sting by the more dangerous species causes marked systemic effects within from 1 to 2 hours, in addition to excruciating pain at the site of the sting. Nausea, vomiting, abdominal pain, shock, convulsions, and coma may develop, and deaths have been recorded.

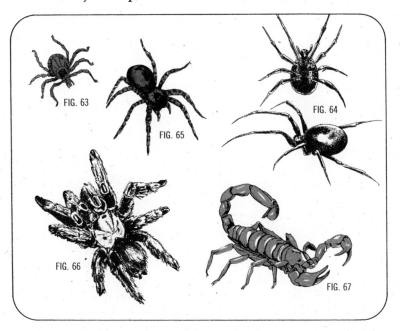

FIG. 63

FIG. 64

FIG. 65

FIG. 66

FIG. 67

First Aid

For Tick Bites

Removal of ticks by using tweezers or by applying heat to them, as with a lighted cigarette, may leave tick parts in the wound or may injure the victim's skin. A better method is to cover the tick with heavy oil (mineral, salad, or machine) to close its breathing pores. It may disengage at once; if not, allow the oil to remain in place for half an hour. Then remove the tick carefully with tweezers, taking time so that all parts are removed.

Gently scrub the area thoroughly with soap and water, because the tick may have left disease germs on the skin.

For Minor Bites and Stings

Use cold applications and soothing lotions, such as calamine.

For Severe Reactions

Administer artificial respiration, if it is warranted.

Apply a constricting band (see Fig. 73, page 116) above the injection site on the victim's arm or leg (between the site and his heart) to slow the absorption of poison that reaches the general circulation of the body. Do not apply the band so tightly that the pulse below it disappears or so that it produces a throbbing sensation. You should be able to slip your index finger under the band when it is in place. Keep the affected part down, below the level of the victim's heart. If medical care is readily available, leave the band in place; otherwise, remove it after 30 minutes.

Apply ice contained in a towel or plastic bag or cold cloths to the site of the sting or bite.

Give a home medication, such as aspirin, for the relief of pain.

In the case of a bee sting, remove and discard the stinger and venom sac.

If the victim has a history of allergic reactions to insect bites or is subject to hay fever or asthma, or if he is not promptly relieved of symptoms, call a physician or take the victim immediately to the nearest source of medical treatment. In the case of a highly sensitive person, do not wait for symptoms to appear—delay can be fatal.

POISONING BY VENOMOUS SNAKES

Kinds and Effects

There are four kinds of poisonous snakes in the United States: rattlesnakes (Fig. 68), copperheads (Fig. 69), cottonmouth moccasins (Fig. 70), and coral snakes (Fig. 71). The first three are called pit vipers (Crotalus species). Each has a pit between the eye and the nostril on each side of the head, elliptical pupils, two well-developed fangs, and one row of plates beneath its tail.

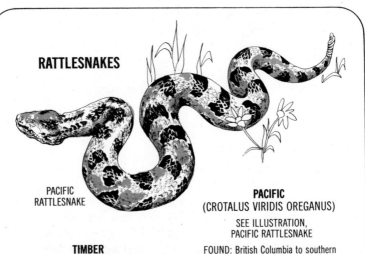

RATTLESNAKES

PACIFIC RATTLESNAKE

PACIFIC
(CROTALUS VIRIDIS OREGANUS)

SEE ILLUSTRATION,
PACIFIC RATTLESNAKE

FOUND: British Columbia to southern
California and lower California;
east to Idaho, Nevada, and Arizona.
SIZE: Up to 5 feet.

TIMBER
(CROTALUS HORRIDUS)
ALSO CALLED:
**BANDED RATTLESNAKE, MOUNTAIN
RATTLER, AND BLACK RATTLER**
FOUND: In uplands and mountains from
southern Maine to northern Florida and
westward to central Texas.
SIZE: Up to 6 feet; average 4 feet.

MASSASAUGA
(SISTRURUS CATENATUS)
ALSO CALLED:
PIGMY RATTLESNAKE
FOUND: Western New York and north-
western Pennsylvania; westward to
northeastern Kansas on the south and
southeastern Minnesota on the north.
A subspecies extends into Texas,
Arizona, and Colorado.
SIZE: Up to 3 feet.

DIAMONDBACK
(CROTALUS ADAMANTEUS)
FOUND: From central coast region of
North Carolina; along lower coastal
plain through Florida; westward to
eastern Louisiana.
SIZE: Up to 8 feet.

FIG. 68

The coral snake is a variety of cobra, found along the coast and lowlands of the Southeast and in the southeastern area of the United States. It is small, has tubular fangs, with teeth behind the fangs, and cannot readily attach itself to large surfaces, such as the forearm and the calf. It has some features of nonpoisonous snakes: round pupils and a double row of plates beneath its tail.

It is characterized by red, yellow, and black rings around the body, with the red and yellow adjoining, and *always* has a *black nose.* Its potent venom affects the victim's nervous system, whereas that of a pit viper affects the victim's circulatory system, destroying red blood cells and interfering with blood clotting.

A nonpoisonous snake has round pupils, no fangs or pits, and a double row of plates beneath its tail.

Each year, the poisonous snakebites reported in the United States total about 6,500, with approximately 15 deaths, most of which are

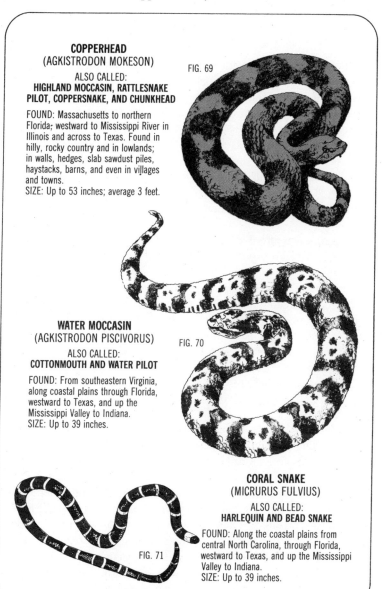

COPPERHEAD
(AGKISTRODON MOKESON)
ALSO CALLED:
HIGHLAND MOCCASIN, RATTLESNAKE PILOT, COPPERSNAKE, AND CHUNKHEAD

FIG. 69

FOUND: Massachusetts to northern Florida; westward to Mississippi River in Illinois and across to Texas. Found in hilly, rocky country and in lowlands; in walls, hedges, slab sawdust piles, haystacks, barns, and even in villages and towns.
SIZE: Up to 53 inches; average 3 feet.

WATER MOCCASIN
(AGKISTRODON PISCIVORUS)
ALSO CALLED:
COTTONMOUTH AND WATER PILOT

FIG. 70

FOUND: From southeastern Virginia, along coastal plains through Florida, westward to Texas, and up the Mississippi Valley to Indiana.
SIZE: Up to 39 inches.

CORAL SNAKE
(MICRURUS FULVIUS)
ALSO CALLED:
HARLEQUIN AND BEAD SNAKE

FIG. 71

FOUND: Along the coastal plains from central North Carolina, through Florida, westward to Texas, and up the Mississippi Valley to Indiana.
SIZE: Up to 39 inches.

caused by rattlesnakes. More than half the bite cases occur in Texas, North Carolina, Florida, Georgia, Louisiana, and Arkansas. Statistics are not available on the number of bites by nonpoisonous snakes or on the effects of first aid or later medical treatment on survival after poisonous snakebite, because the mortality rate is so low. The following conditions influence the severity of both the local and the general reactions:

- The amount of venom injected—This condition depends in part on the kind and size of the snake. For example, the average rattlesnake injects one-third more venom than a water moccasin and five times more than a copperhead. Venom from a coral snake is much more toxic, although usually only a small quantity is injected. Snakes do not, as a rule, inject all their available venom at one strike; if part of the supply has been discharged previously, a smaller amount will be available, and the reaction will be less severe.
- The size of the victim—For example, the reaction in a child is greater.
- The protection afforded by clothing—Includes shoes and gloves.
- The speed of absorption of venom into the circulation—Absorption takes place through the lymphatic channels into the bloodstream, unless venom happens to be injected directly into a vein. The *general* reaction is less if venom is absorbed slowly; the *local* reaction, however, may be increased by measures taken to slow the rate of absorption from the location of the bite.
- The time that passes before the victim receives specific antivenin therapy.
- The location of the bite.

Signs and Symptoms

The bite of a pit viper is extremely painful and is characterized by rapid swelling of the involved area. If only minimal swelling occurs within 30 minutes, the bite will almost certainly have been from a nonpoisonous snake.

A pit viper inflicts one or more puncture wounds, depositing venom beneath the skin, but identification of its fang marks (Fig. 72) is not always possible. When the venom from a pit viper is absorbed, there is general discoloration of the skin due to destruction of red cells and marked pain and swelling. There is general weakness, rapid pulse, and sometimes nausea, shortness of breath, dimness of vision, vomiting, and shock, all of which may come on gradually over a period of from 1 to 2 hours.

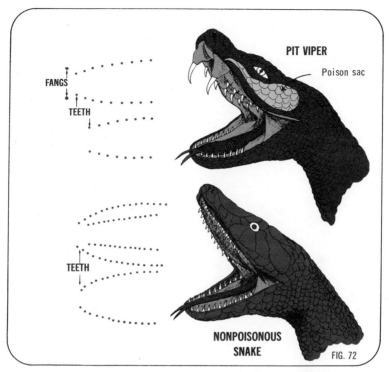

FANGS
TEETH

PIT VIPER
Poison sac

TEETH

NONPOISONOUS
SNAKE
FIG. 72

The venom of a coral snake usually causes only slight burning pain and mild swelling at the wound but it is extremely toxic. The nerve toxin of a coral snake may or may not result in burning pain and local swelling but it does produce blurring vision, drooping eyelids, slurring speech, drowsiness, and increased salivation and sweating. Nausea and vomiting, shock, respiratory difficulty, paralysis, convulsions, and coma may develop. All reactions from snakebite are aggravated by acute fear and anxiety.

First Aid

The objectives of first aid for snakebites are to reduce the circulation of blood through the bite area, to delay absorption of venom, to prevent aggravation of the local wound, and to sustain respiration.

The victim should not be permitted to walk or to move involved body parts. He should be reassured continuously. He should be taken to a source of medical assistance as quickly as possible.

- Immobilize the victim's arm or leg in the lowered position, keeping the involved area *below* the level of his heart.

- If the bite is on the arm or leg, apply a constricting band (Fig. 73) from 2 to 4 inches above the bite, between the wound and the victim's heart, to decrease the flow of lymph from the affected area. The constricting band should be snug but loose enough to allow blood to flow into the limb. If the band is properly adjusted, there will be some oozing from the wound.

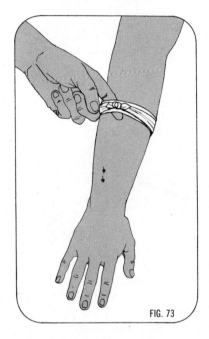

FIG. 73

- Use the blade in a snakebite kit, if available; otherwise, sterilize a knife blade with a flame, and make incisions through the skin at each fang mark and over the suspected venom deposit point. (The snake strikes downward, and the deposit point will be lower than the fang marks.) Be very careful to make the incisions through the skin only and in the long axis of the limb. Do *not* make cross-cut incisions. The incisions must not be deeper than the skin because of the danger of severing muscles and nerves. Special care is necessary in making incisions on the hand, wrist, or foot, because muscles, nerves, and tendons lie close to the surface, and the injury may cause considerable disability. Do not make incisions more than one-half inch long.
- Apply suction with the suction cup contained in the snakebite kit, if available; otherwise, use your mouth. Snake venom is not a stomach poison but it should not be swallowed, and you should

rinse it from your mouth. Continue suction for from 30 to 60 minutes. If swelling extends up to the constricting band, apply another band a few inches above the first, but leave the first band in place.

- Wash the wound thoroughly with soap and water and blot it dry.
- Apply a sterile or clean dressing and bandage it in place.
- You may place a cold, wet cloth or ice wrapped in a cloth, if available, over the wound to slow absorption. *Do not pack the wound in ice.*
- Do not give the victim alcohol in any form. Alcohol dilates blood vessels of the skin and increases absorption.
- Treat the victim for shock. You may give him sips of fluid if he is conscious and can swallow without difficulty, unless nausea and vomiting develop.
- Watch for any sign of breathing difficulty, especially after a coral snake bite. Give the victim artificial respiration, if it is warranted.
- Even if the bite has been inflicted by a nonpoisonous snake, a physician should be consulted with regard to antibiotic therapy and prevention of tetanus.
- If the victim is without help and must walk, he should move slowly.

Telephone ahead to the nearest hospital or physician so that antivenin can quickly be made available. Administration of antivenin is not a first aid procedure; it requires preliminary testing of the victim for sensitivity to horse serum. Only a person with medical training should attempt to give the antivenin.

Death from snakebite rarely occurs immediately; most often, it occurs within from 1 to 2 days after injury. The tissue at the site of the wound often sloughs away, leaving a large, raw ulcer that may later require skin grafting or some other type of reconstructive surgery. Many surgeons excise the area of the bite as soon as possible after injury to remove venom-containing tissues and avoid gangrene.

8

DRUGS AND THEIR ABUSE

Administered under medical direction, drugs often appear to have miraculous effects in relieving suffering, combating disease, and saving life. When the same drugs are misused or abused, they can become deadly enemies.

DEFINITIONS

A drug is a substance that affects the functions of the body or mind when taken into the body or applied to its surface. Some drugs are readily available and are sold over the counter as home remedies. Most drugs, however, are subject to some control or regulation for the protection of health and the promotion of well-being. These drugs are available only on a physician's prescription and are intended to be administered only under the direction of a physician. Such use of drugs constitutes accepted medical practice.

Note that the word *drug* is defined broadly here and is not synonomous with the word *medicament*. Abuse of some substances that are not used in medical practice but are drugs by definition may be particularly widespread and hazardous.

Drug misuse is the use of drugs for—

- Purposes or conditions for which they are unsuited
- Appropriate purposes but in improper dosage

Drug abuse is the excessive or persistent use of a drug without regard to accepted medical practice.

Drug dependence is the condition that results from drug abuse. It is described as the interaction between the drug and the body when this interaction involves an effect on the central nervous system. It is characterized by a behavioral response that always includes a compulsive desire to continue taking the drug, either to experience its effects or to avoid the discomfort of its absence. Dependence always involves psychic craving (psychic dependence) and sometimes involves physical, organic disturbance (physical dependence).

IDENTIFICATION OF DRUG ABUSE

Almost any drug can be misused or abused. Some drugs are commonly abused, constituting personal and public health problems, with social, economic, and legal implications.

In cases of drug abuse emergency, it is important that the signs and symptoms of the abuse are identified by the person providing the immediate assistance. The type and amount of substance used and the time it was taken should be determined, if possible. When the drugs have been taken by mouth and if the individual is seen at the time of oral ingestion or within a few minutes afterward, an effort to empty the stomach to prevent absorption is recommended.

It is sometimes difficult to distinguish between types of drugs taken merely by observing symptoms. This difficulty is increased when drugs are used in combination. The necessary clues to identification are often provided by apparatus, such as teaspoons, paper packs, eye droppers, hypodermic needles, vials, or collapsible tubes. The presence of gelatin capsules, pills, or other drug containers, or of needle marks (Fig. 74) on a victim's body is also significant and should be noted.

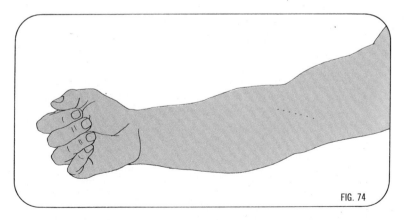

FIG. 74

Information on the types of drugs taken, plus information on the age and size of the victim and his general condition and behavior, should be provided to the drug abuse center or the attending physician.

CLASSIFICATION OF DRUGS

Drugs that are abused can be classified in many ways. Some of the groups overlap in one or more effects. The following list is arranged for convenience, without regard to importance, severity, or prevalence of abuse:

- Alcohol (alcoholic beverages)
- Cannabis (marihuana)
- Depressants (sedatives-hypnotics)
- Hallucinogens
- Inhalants
- Narcotics
- Stimulants
- Tranquilizers

Alcohol

In this context, the term *alcohol* refers to alcoholic beverages, whose effects are related to their alcoholic content and to the level of alcohol in the blood resulting from their use. The use of alcohol is legal and widely accepted socially in the United States and in many other countries. In spite of this acceptance, prolonged abuse and consumption of large amounts of alcohol may cause great social and economic detriment, as well as physical damage to the individual users.

Even a moderate amount of alcohol in combination with a barbiturate or minor tranquilizer may be hazardous.

Effects

Alcohol is a depressant, affecting first the higher reasoning areas of the brain, with perhaps a feeling of relaxation or, in the company of others, a sense of exhilaration and conviviality due to the release of inhibitions. Later, motor activity, motor skills, and coordination are disrupted, and, with deepening intoxication, other bodily processes are disturbed. In the most severe stages of alcohol intoxication, superficial blood vessels are dilated, causing a feeling of warmth, even though the actual effect is an increased loss of body heat. Respiration decreases, consciousness wanes, and coma and death may result.

Abuse

The drinker may use alcohol as a psychological crutch. Thus, he may develop a psychic, and later a physical, dependence similar to that produced by the barbiturates. There is a well-defined abstinence syndrome closely related to that described for the barbiturates. Delirium tremens is a major symptom complex of alcohol withdrawal.

The odor of alcohol on a person's breath does not necessarily indicate intoxication. In addition to the noting of information on incoordination, disturbance of speech, and altered respiration, other means are commonly used to determine whether the level of alcohol in the body equals or exceeds that of legally defined intoxication. The drinker is often unaware of detriment to his normal skills and should be restrained from activity requiring such skills, particularly driving.

First Aid

Alcohol intoxication, whether due to an acute overdose or to prolonged abuse, is treated as follows:

- If the person is sleeping quietly, his face is of normal color, his breathing is normal, and his pulse is regular, no immediate first aid is necessary.
- If the person shows such signs of shock as cold and clammy skin, rapid and thready pulse, and abnormal breathing, or if he does not respond at all, obtain medical aid immediately.
- Maintain an open airway, give artificial respiration, if indicated, and maintain body heat.
- If the victim is unconscious, place him in the coma position (Fig. 75) so that secretions may drool from his mouth. This position will usually allow for good respiration.
- Remember that an intoxicated person may be violent and obstreperous and will need careful handling to prevent him from harming himself and others.

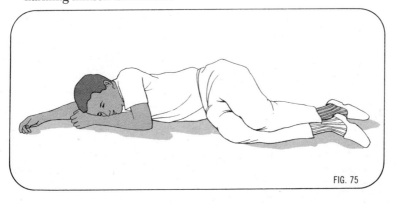

FIG. 75

The alcoholic should be encouraged to seek help from Alcoholics Anonymous or from a drug abuse treatment center.

Cannabis (Marihuana)

Cannabis sativa is an herbaceous annual plant that grows wild in temperate climates in many parts of the world. The various forms of the drug are frequently referred to as cannabis, although the official definition states that cannabis is "the flowering or fruiting tops of the cannabis plant from which the resin has not been extracted." Marihuana usually consists of crushed cannabis leaves and flowers, and often twigs. It varies greatly in the content of active material. Hashish is a preparation of cannabis resin, which is squeezed or scraped from the plant top and is generally five or more times as potent as marihuana. Marihuana is smoked; hashish may be smoked but is also commonly made into a confection or beverage.

Effects

The use of cannabis in medical practice is not presently recognized. The effects to be described, therefore, are those experienced in abuse. These effects are dose-related; that is, the effects are dependent upon the content of active material—tetrahydrocannabinols, in particular. The impression that marihuana is a harmless drug has been fostered by the low content of active material in American samples; however, use of the more potent hashish is increasing.

The *immediate physical effects* of smoking one or more marihuana cigarettes include—

Throat irritation
Increased heart rate
Reddening of the eyes
Occasional dizziness, incoordination, or sleepiness
Increased appetite

The *psychological effects* vary from individual to individual and with the amount of the drug taken. Among the effects described are feelings of exhilaration, hilarity, and conviviality, but there is also distortion of time and space perception, and there may be disturbance of psychomotor activity, which would impair driving and other skills.

In some individuals and in connection with excessive use of the drug, a psychotoxic reaction resembling a "bad trip" on LSD may occur.

Many persons try marihuana once or twice and then abandon it; some use it intermittently—usually in the company of others—and many use it continually. Marihuana can produce psychic dependence, but there is no evidence of physical dependence, and no withdrawal symptoms follow discontinuance.

First Aid

There is no need for emergency treatment unless a psychotoxic reaction develops, in which case the approach is the same as that for a bad LSD trip.

Depressants (Sedatives-Hypnotics)

Depressants (downers) are drugs that act on the nervous system, promoting relaxation and sleep. Chief among these drugs are the barbiturates, the more important of which are—

Phenobarbital (goofballs)
Pentobarbital (yellow jackets)
Amobarbital (blue devils)
Secobarbital (red devils)

Closely related are the nonbarbiturate sedatives, some of which are—

Glutethimide (Doriden)
Chloral hydrate (knockout drops)
Paraldehyde

Effects

A usual therapeutic dose of a barbiturate does not relieve pain but has a calming, relaxing effect that promotes sleep. Reactions include—

Relief of anxiety and excitement
Tendency to reduce mental and physical activity
Slight decrease in breathing

Barbiturates are used to reduce the frequency of convulsions in epileptics, and one in particular—Pentothal—is given intravenously as a preoperative sedative.

An overdose of barbiturates produces unconsciousness, deepening to a coma, from which the victim cannot be roused. Barbiturates are frequently involved in instances of accidental or intentional suicide.

Some accidental poisonings occur when a person becomes confused, as a dose of barbiturates starts to take effect, and inadvertently takes a second dose. Another cause of accidental poisoning is the mutual enhancement of effect that takes place when a barbiturate is taken in conjunction with alcohol. This combination can be lethal, even in small amounts.

Abuse

Barbiturates are commonly abused in two ways:

- The barbiturate is taken in increasing amounts by persons who have developed tolerance to the drug, and thus require larger and larger doses to feel the desired effects
- For a thrill, the barbiturate is injected as an alternate to other drugs that are being abused, particularly amphetamines. Barbiturates can produce dependence, both psychic and physical.

Abrupt discontinuance of barbiturate administration to the dependent person causes the following characteristic withdrawal symptoms:

Restlessness, insomnia, and tremors
Muscular twitching
Nausea and vomiting
Convulsions
Delusions and hallucinations

The convulsions and the psychotic symptoms seldom occur at the same time. The convulsions are likely to occur on the second or third day of withdrawal, the delusions and hallucinations a little later. The other symptoms usually occur within 24 hours of withdrawal. If the individual is not treated, the symptoms last about a week. Abrupt withdrawal of barbiturates is dangerous. Withdrawal should take place gradually and under medical supervision. The dependent person should be persuaded to get help from a physician or a drug abuse treatment center.

First Aid

- Maintain an open airway and give the victim artificial respiration, if indicated.
- Maintain body temperature.
- Get the victim to a physician or hospital as soon as possible.

Hallucinogens

Hallucinogens are drugs that are capable of producing mood changes, frequently of a bizarre character; disturbances of sensation, thought, emotion, and self-awareness; alteration of time and space perception; and both illusions and delusions. The most important hallucinogen is lysergic acid diethylamide (LSD). Some others are—

Mescaline
Psilocybin
Morning glory seeds
A number of synthetic substances

Since none of these substances presently has accepted medical use, the effects to be described are those experienced in abuse.

Effects

Abuse of hallucinogens is of the spree type: the drug is taken intermittently, although perhaps as often as several times a week. Many persons develop a psychic drive for repetition of the experience, but physical dependence does not develop. The effects may often seem pleasurable and rewarding but they may also be very unpleasant (a "bad trip"), even in the same individual.

LSD, for example, is likely to produce these physical effects:

Increased activity through its action on the central nervous system
Increased heart rate
Increased blood pressure
Increased body temperature
Dilated (enlarged) pupils (see page 126, Fig. 76)
Flushed face

The psychological effects of hallucinogens, in general, are highly variable and unpredictable. They include an emergence into consciousness of previously suppressed ideas, strong emotional feeling, an impression of astonishingly lucid thought, a feeling of insight and creativity, and an intensification of sensory impressions. Changes in sensation may also be involved (sounds are seen, ordinary things appear beautiful, colors seem to be heard. A feeling of cosmic oneness, profound religious awareness, and a mood of joy and peace may also mark the use of the hallucinogens.

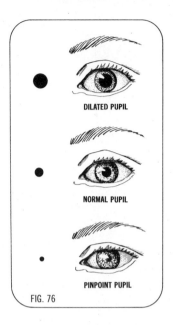

FIG. 76

In the bad trip, or "freak-out," there is an intense experience of fear, or nightmarish terror to the point of panic. Other undesirable effects are—

Complete loss of emotional control
Paranoid delusions
Hallucinations
Profound depression
Tension and anxiety

Disordered social behavior may also occur. Because of the delusions and disordered sensations, the user may think he is immune to harm, or perhaps able to fly, and may suffer severe physical injury. Flashbacks (sensory replays of previous "trips") are associated with the use of hallucinogenic drugs such as LSD, and such flashbacks may occur months after the drug has been taken. They may be severe or simply amount to a feeling of dizziness or a temporary blackout.

First Aid

- A person on a "trip," good or bad, needs careful attention, reassurance, and protection from bodily harm or the results of his antisocial behavior.

- Talk the person down from his disturbing experience in quiet and safe surroundings.
- Get the victim to a physician or hospital as soon as possible. Two persons should accompany him, if possible.

Inhalants

Occasional self-administration of volatile substances such as ether or chloroform in order to experience intoxication is a very old practice. In recent years, inhalation of a wide variety of substances, a practice commonly referred to as glue-sniffing, has become widespread among young people in their early teens. The substances inhaled include—

Fast-drying glue or cement (such as model airplane glue)
Many paints and lacquers and their thinners and removers
Gasoline
Kerosene
Lighter fluid and dry-cleaning fluid
Nail polish and remover

The usual methods of inhaling are to hold a cloth over the nose and mouth with some of the substance on it or to cover the head with a paper or plastic bag containing a quantity of the substance.

Effects

The effects resulting from the use of inhalants are those experienced in abuse. Reactions are—

Initial excitement resulting from release of inhibitions
Irritation of the respiratory passages
Unsteadiness
Drunkenness, with growing depression that deepens even to unconsciousness

A serious potential danger accompanies waning consciousness in a person who uses a bag over his head for inhaling: Failure to remove the bag from the inhaler's head may result in suffocation.

Some of the propellants in the aerosols that are inhaled are toxic to the heart and can cause death by alteration in the rhythm of the heartbeat. This situation requires prompt and intensive medical attention. Persistent use of inhalants may cause some psychic dependence and may produce pathological changes in the liver and other organs.

First Aid

- If a person is found with a bag or other apparatus over his head, remove it immediately.
- If breathing stops, administer artificial respiration.
- Obtain medical assistance immediately.

Narcotics

"Narcotics" refers, in general, to opium and specifically to—

Preparations of opium, such as paregoric.
Substances found in opium (morphine and codeine).
Substances derived from morphine (heroin, Dilaudid, etc.).
Synthetic (laboratory-made) substances that have morphine-like effects, including merperidine or Demerol, methadone or Dolophine.

In late 1970, federal laws governing the control of narcotics appropriately excluded cocaine and marihuana from the narcotics classification. Cocaine is a stimulant that affects the central nervous system, and marihuana is a mood- and sense-altering substance.

Effects

A therapeutic dose of a narcotic relieves pain and reaction to pain, calms anxiety, and promotes sleep. Common reactions to morphine, heroin, and other morphinelike agents include—

Reduction in awareness of pain
Quieting of tension and anxiety
Decrease in activity
Promotion of sleep
Decrease in breathing and pulse rate
Reduction of hunger and thirst
Some unpleasant reactions to narcotics include sweating, dizziness, nausea, vomiting, and constipation.

An overdose of a narcotic results in—
Lethargy and increasing reduction in activity and awareness
Sleep, deepening to coma (prolonged unconsciousness)
Increasing depression of breathing to the point of respiratory failure
Profuse sweating

Fall in temperature
Muscle relaxation
Contraction of pupils to pinpoint size (See Fig. 76, page 126.)
except with meperidine

Abuse

The continued administration of a narcotic produces both psychic and physical dependence. Discontinuing the drug causes the appearance of the characteristic, recognizable, withdrawal symptoms within from 6 to 24 hours. The symptoms and signs include—

Nervousness, restlessness, and anxiety
Tears and a running nose
Sweating, hot and cold flashes, and gooseflesh
Yawning
Muscular aches and pains in legs, back, and abdomen
Nausea, vomiting, and diarrhea (uncontrollable and continuous)
Loss of appetite and loss of weight
Dilated (enlarged) pupils (See Fig. 76, page 126.)
Increased breathing, blood pressure, and body temperature
Intense craving for the drug (for a "fix")

If withdrawal symptoms are in evidence they may be promptly relieved by a dose of the same drug or of another drug in the same group. There is little the lay person can do for the individual in withdrawal except to reassure him and to persuade him to go to a drug treatment center or a physician. Other problems associated with the abuse of narcotics are infection, resulting from the use of unsterile needles, the possibility of developing hepatitis, and malnutrition and dental caries (decay) due to neglect of dietary and hygienic practices.

First Aid

- Arouse the victim, if possible, by lightly slapping him with a cold, wet towel, and try to get him on his feet.
- Maintain an open airway and administer artificial respiration if indicated.
- Maintain body temperature.
- Avoid rough treatment of the victim.
- Reassure the victim and seek medical assistance as soon as possible.

Stimulants

Stimulants (uppers) are used to increase mental activity and to offset drowsiness and fatigue. The most commonly abused stimulants are—

Amphetamine (Benzedrine—bennies, pep pills)
Dextroamphetamine (Dexedrine—dexies)
Methamphetamine (Methedrine—meth, speed, crystal)
Methylphenidate (Ritalin)

All of these act similarly and will be described as exemplified by amphetamine.

Caffeine and cocaine are included among the stimulants. Caffeine is a constituent of coffee, tea, and other beverages. It may produce a very mild psychic dependence but it does not cause personal or social damage. Cocaine, used medically as a local anesthetic, is a powerful central nervous system stimulant.

Effects

A therapeutic dose of amphetamine produces the following effects:

Alertness
Wakefulness
Relief from fatigue
A feeling of well-being

Mental and physical performance may increase to some extent.

Amphetamine reduces hunger and has been widely used for this purpose, although the effect is not well sustained, and the feelings of alertness and wakefulness wear off. Amphetamine increases blood pressure, breathing rate, and general bodily activity. Tolerance to the effects of amphetamine can develop to a high degree, resulting in a demand for increased doses.

An overdose of amphetamine may produce toxic effects when taken orally, but these effects are more common when amphetamine is taken by intravenous injection. Use of amphetamines as antiobesity agents (diet pills) has limited value, and there is little recognized medical need for these drugs, although they are occasionally used in treating narcolepsy (uncontrollable desire for sleep) or hyperkinetic (overactive) states.

Abuse

Amphetamine abuse can produce strong psychic dependence and a pronounced degree of tolerance, but not physical dependence.

Prolonged administration of oral doses for diet or fatigue control, because of the accompanying sense of well-being, frequently leads to abuse when the doses are increased in an effort to maintain an effect. This abuse produces a psychic dependence on the drug, but withdrawal should be possible without serious incident.

In recent years, a form of amphetamine abuse involving repeated intravenous injection of the drug (usually Methedrine or Dexedrine) has developed. Called a "speed run," this abuse is accompanied by considerable risk to the user and the people around him. The pattern of abuse begins with several days of repeated injections, which increase in size and frequency. The daily total sometimes reaches more than 100 times the initial dose. At first, the user may feel energetic, talkative, enthusiastic, happy, and confident. He does not sleep and usually eats little or nothing. After a few days, unpleasant symptoms appear and increase as the dosage increases. These symptoms include—

Confusion
Disorganization
Compulsive repetition of small, meaningless acts
Irritability
Suspiciousness
Fear
Hallucinations and delusions, which may become paranoid
Aggressive and antisocial behavior, which may endanger others

The run, which usually lasts less than a week, is abruptly terminated. The abuser is left exhausted. He sleeps—sometimes for several days—and upon awakening, he is emotionally depressed, lethargic, and extremely hungry. Shortly, another run is begun, and the cycle is repeated. There is little that can be done for the victim except to protect him against injury and to seek psychiatric help for him for his delusions and hallucinations.

Abuse of cocaine may take a form similar to the speed run, with rapid, repeated intravenous injections followed by psychotoxic symptoms similar to those characteristic of amphetamine, particularly delusions of a paranoid nature. Another cocaine abuse practice is the taking of the drug alternately or concurrently with heroin. In combination, cocaine provides the "up" and heroin the "down."

Cocaine abuse results in strong psychic dependence but not physical dependence.

First Aid

- Protect the victim against injury.
- Maintain an open airway, and administer artificial respiration if indicated.
- Maintain body temperature.
- Obtain psychiatric help for the victim for his delusions and hallucinations.

Tranquilizers

Types and Abuse

Agents in this category are commonly referred to as major and minor tranquilizers.

The major tranquilizers include the phenothiazines (chlorpromazine, for example) and reserpine. They are used in treating mental disease to calm psychotic patients. They have not produced dependence, but overdosage of these drugs produces a deepening state of unconsciousness, a fall in body temperature and blood pressure, and eventual respiratory failure. The effects produced by an overdose are prolonged, and the victim must be watched carefully as long as severe central nervous system depression persists

The minor tranquilizers are used to calm anxiety and other feelings of stress and excitement without producing sleep. At high dose levels, their effects are virtually indistinguishable from the effects of the sedative hypnotics. Common examples of minor tranquilizers are—

Meprobamate (Miltown, Equanil)
Chlordiazepoxide (Librium)
Ethchlorvynol (Placidyl)
Diazepam (Valium)

Some tranquilizers are used in treating chronic alcoholism, but in effect this usage represents substitution of one depressant drug for another. These drugs are useful in treating acute alcohol withdrawal.

Prolonged administration of a minor tranquilizer, with a tendency to increase the dose, may result in psychic and physical dependence. The characteristics of dependence on minor tranquilizers and the related withdrawal symptoms are similar to those produced by barbiturates.

First Aid

- Arouse the victim, if possible, by lightly slapping him with a cold, wet towel and try to get him on his feet.
- Maintain an open airway and apply artificial respiration if indicated.
- Maintain body temperature.
- Get the victim to a physician, hospital, or drug abuse treatment center as soon as possible.

9

BURNS

Burns are a leading cause of accidental death in the United States. Every year, approximately 8,000 persons lose their lives in fires—half of them under 14 years old or over 64 years old. Often, several members of a family are burned to death at the same time. All too often, small children left at home unattended are burned to death.

Property damage from fire is enormous: almost a half billion dollars a year from a total of over 800,000 fires. The impact on family members from the loss of their home can seldom be realized, especially if prolonged loss of income and the cost of medical care are added to it.

DEFINITION

A burn is an injury that results from heat, chemical agents, or radiation. It may vary in depth, size, and severity and may damage cells in the affected area.

CAUSES AND EFFECTS

Burns are caused most commonly by carelessness with matches and cigarettes; scalds from hot liquids; defective heating, cooking, and electrical equipment; use of open fires that produce flame burns, especially when flammable clothing is worn; unsafe practices in the home in the use of flammable liquids for starting fires and for cleaning and scrubbing wax off floors; immersion in overheated bath water; and use of such chemicals as lye, strong acids, and strong detergents.

In addition to surface burns and the effects of heat on the blood and on body tissues other than the skin, the hazards of fire include the following:

- Inhalation of very hot (superheated) air or irritating or poisonous gases, including carbon monoxide.
- Asphyxia from insufficient oxygen in the air.
- Falls and injuries from collapsing walls in burning buildings.

In burns of large areas of the body surface, loss of plasma and changes in the balance of fluids and chemicals in the body contribute to the development of shock.

CLASSIFICATION

Burns are usually classified by depth or degree. When a burn is first examined, classification may be difficult or impossible. The most reliable guide is the causative agent, but often the degree will differ in various parts of the same affected area.

First Degree

The usual signs of first-degree burns (Fig. 77) are redness or discoloration, mild swelling, and pain. Healing occurs rapidly. First-degree burns result from overexposure to the sun, light contact with hot objects, and scalding by hot water or steam.

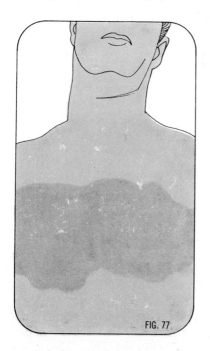

FIG. 77

Second Degree

Second-degree burns (Fig. 78) are deeper than first-degree burns and appear red or mottled, with blister formation. There is considerable swelling over a period of several days and, as a rule, a wet surface due to loss of plasma through the damaged layers of the skin. This type of injury results from very deep sunburn, contact with hot liquids, and flash burns from gasoline, kerosene, and other products. Second-degree burns are usually more painful than deepèr ones, since in third-degree burns, the nerve endings in the skin are destroyed.

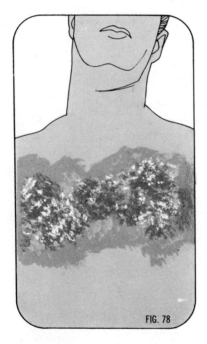

FIG. 78

Third Degree

Third-degree burns (Fig. 79) involve deeper destruction. A burn may look white or charred or at first may resemble a second-degree burn. In both third-degree and deep second-degree burns, there is coagulation of the skin and destruction of red blood cells. Third-degree burns can be caused by flame, ignited clothing, immersion in hot water, contact with hot objects, or electricity.

Many burns are a combination of first-, second-, and third-degree burns, with patchy involvement, and nearly all full-thickness (third-

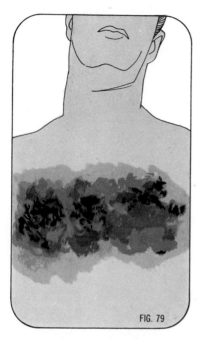

FIG. 79

degree) burns are surrounded by areas of less involvement. Because determining the depth of a burn by inspection alone is usually impossible, knowledge of the circumstances of the injury is very important. Temperature and duration of contact, in particular, are important factors in determining how much tissue has been destroyed.

In both first-degree and second-degree burns, only a partial thickness of the skin is involved, and new skin will grow if serious infection does not develop. In third-degree burns, which involve complete loss of all layers of the skin and at times involve the deeper structures, true skin healing cannot take place except at the margins of the wound, and scar tissue replaces the rest of the area.

EXTENT AND LOCATION

In addition to classification according to depth, or degree, burns are ordinarily described according to the extent of the total body surface involved (Fig. 80)—for example, 40 percent total burn with 20 percent third-degree or full-thickness. Calculations of the extent of burns are often difficult, even for physicians.

In general, an adult who has suffered burns of 15 percent of his body surface (a child, 10 percent), wherever located, requires hospi-

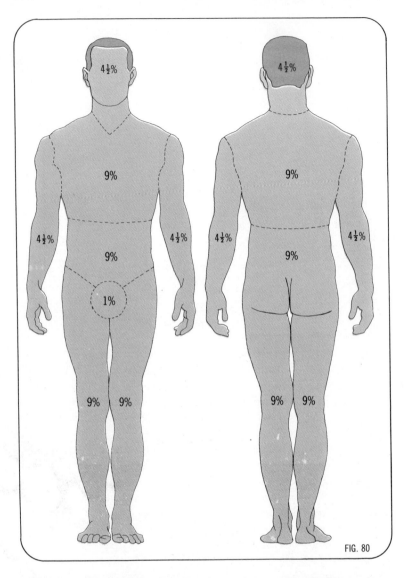

FIG. 80

talization. Burns of the hands, feet, or face also should receive prompt medical attention. Burns of the face are often associated with injury to the respiratory tract and may lead to obstruction of breathing as swelling increases. Persons with third-degree burns of 50 percent or more of the body surface have an extremely high mortality rate. For persons over 60 years old, third-degree burns of even 30 percent carry great risk as far as survival is concerned.

FIRST AID

The objectives of first aid for burns are to relieve pain, prevent contamination, and treat for shock.

First Degree

Medical treatment is usually not required. To relieve pain, apply cold water applications to the affected area or submerge the burned area in cold water (Fig. 81). A dry dressing may be applied if desired.

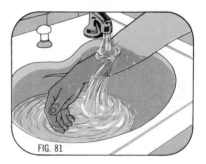

FIG. 81

Second Degree (Small)

Immerse the burned parts in cold water (not ice water) or apply freshly ironed or laundered cloths that have been wrung out in ice water until the pain subsides. Immediate cooling can reduce the burning effect of heat in the deeper layers of skin. Never add salt to ice water; it lowers the temperature and may produce further injury. Gently blot the area dry with sterile gauze, a clean cloth, a towel, or other household linen. Do not use absorbent cotton. Apply dry, sterile gauze or clean cloth as a protective dressing. Do not try to break blisters or remove shreds of tissue, and do not use an antiseptic preparation, ointment, spray, or home remedy on a severe burn.

If there must be a delay in getting medical attention, leave the dressing in place for 4 or 5 days, unless it becomes soaked with exudate or develops an unpleasant odor. If removal of the dressing becomes necessary, rinse the area with large amounts of water to free the dressing from the surface of the burn. Wash the area gently with a mild soap and water. Blot it dry with sterile or clean towels before applying a new dressing.

If arms or legs are affected, they should be kept elevated. Every effort should be made to keep the victim from exerting pressure for long periods on burned areas of the back, elbows, legs, and heels. Bed rest is *essential* if the legs and feet are involved, even if the burns are small, because healing is considerably delayed in all wounds of the legs and feet.

Second Degree (Extensive)

Second-degree burns that cover 15 percent or more of the body surface in adults (10 percent or more in children) require hospitalization of the victim, but any *deep second-degree burn* of the hand, foot, or face requires prompt medical care as well. First aid for extensive second-degree burns is the same as for third-degree burns.

Third Degree

Do not remove adhered particles of charred clothing. Cover the burned areas with a sterile dressing or a freshly ironed or laundered sheet or other household linen.

If the victim's *hands* are involved, keep them higher than his heart. They may be held in a vertical position or may be supported on pillows if the victim is lying down.

Burned *feet* or *legs* should be elevated. The victim should not be allowed to walk.

Persons with *face* burns should sit up or be propped up and should be under continuous observation for breathing difficulty. If respiratory problems develop, keep the airway open. It may be necessary to use the *back* of a spoon or similar object to hold the victim's tongue down while his head is tilted back, but care must be taken not to induce vomiting. If possible, his chin should be brought upward and forward.

Transportation to the hospital should be arranged as quickly as possible. If medical help or trained ambulance personnel will not reach the scene for an hour or more and if the victim is *conscious* and *not vomiting*, give him a weak solution of salt and soda at home or en route (1 level teaspoonful salt and 1/2 level teaspoonful baking soda in each quart of water, neither hot nor cold). Do not give alcoholic beverages. Allow the victim to sip slowly. Give an adult about 4 ounces (a half glass) over a period of 15 minutes; give a child from 1 to 12 years old about 2 ounces; and give an infant, under 1 year old, about 1 ounce. Discontinue fluids if vomiting occurs. Fluid may be given by mouth *only* if medical help will not be available for an hour or more and is not otherwise contraindicated.

Aspirin or other home medication may be given for pain, but remember that burn victims are anxious and fearful and need frequent reassurance more than they need drugs for pain.

Do not apply ice water over an extensive burned area, because cold may intensify the shock reaction. However, a cold pack may be applied to a burned face or to burned hands or feet. Do not add salt to the water and do not immerse the burned parts in ice water. Do not apply ointment, commercial burn preparation, grease, or other home remedy. These may cause complications and interfere with treatment by the physician.

Chemical Burns

When irritating chemicals come into contact with the skin or mucous membrane, injury usually begins instantly, and first aid should be immediate. Among such chemicals are acids and alkalis, or corrosive chemicals. Chemical burns are the same as burns caused by flame, steam, or hot liquids.

The essential first aid is to wash away the chemical completely, as quickly as possible, with large quantities of water, using a shower or a hose if available (Fig. 82). Immediate washing is more important

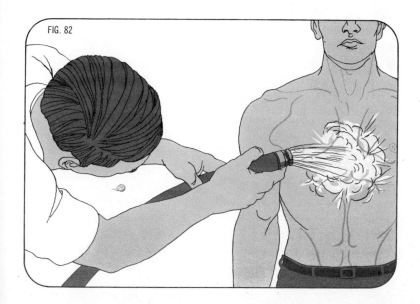

FIG. 82

than neutralizing the chemical and should be continued for at least 5 minutes. Remove the victim's clothing from the areas involved.

- If first aid directions for burns caused by specific chemicals are available (e.g., on a label), follow them.
- You may use rubbing alcohol as a final rinse in carbolic acid burns of the skin.
- You may use a weak solution of vinegar and water as a final rinse in alkali burns.
- Do not use rubbing alcohol or vinegar in the victim's eyes.
- After removing the chemical by washing, give additional first aid as for burns caused by heat.

Burns of the Eye

Acid Burns

First aid for acid burns of the eye should begin as quickly as possible with washing of the face, eyelids, and eye thoroughly with water (Figs. 83 and 84) for at least 5 minutes. Make sure the

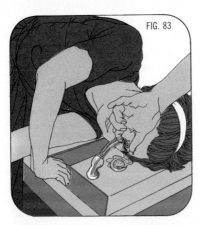
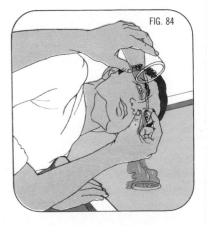

chemical does not wash into the other eye. If the victim is lying down, turn his head to the side and pour the water from the inner corner of his eye outward, holding his eyelids open. If you can quickly make a weak soda solution (1 teaspoonful of baking soda added to 1 quart of water), do so and use it, but begin by washing the eye with tap water.

- Call a physician as quickly as possible and ask for advice.
- Cover the eye with a dry, clean, protective dressing. Do not use absorbent cotton, because fibers may enter the eye. Caution the victim against rubbing his eye, because rubbing might cause further injury.
- Give home remedies for pain, such as aspirin, if necessary.
- Take the victim to an eye specialist; if this is not possible or if one is not available, get other medical assistance.

Alkali Burns

Alkali burns of the eye result in penetrating, progressive injuries, and an eye that first appears to have only slight surface injury may develop deep inflammation and tissue destruction, with loss of vision. Injuries to the eyes from strong laundry and dishwasher detergents and other cleaning solutions used in the home are becoming frequent. Splashing these alkali products into the eyes or rubbing the eyes when using such products may result in serious injury. First aid should be carried out as described previously for acid burns, with the following exceptions:

- After rapidly washing the victim's face, eyelid, and eye with tap water, hold the lids open and continue irrigation for at least 15 minutes.
- Meanwhile, if particles of dry chemicals are floating on the eye, lift them off gently with sterile gauze, a clean handkerchief, or a folded, dry facial tissue (Fig. 85).
- Do not irrigate the eye with soda solution.

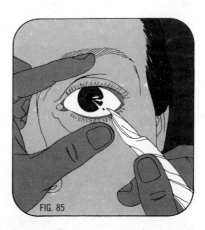

FIG. 85

Irritating Gases

Eye injuries caused by irritating gases are common, and lung damage may result also if a sufficient quantity is involved (see chapter 7, page 102). Many drugs and chemicals are used in spray form. Tear gas in concentrated form may cause blindness and should be handled carefully. Exposure to ammonia, sulfur dioxide, or other gases used in refrigeration may produce severe alkali burns. Sulfur dioxide is particularly dangerous, in that it may cause delayed injury after several hours unless first aid is administered. First aid for eye injuries caused by gases consists of irrigation of the eyes with large quantities of water.

Sunburn

Sunburn is produced primarily by exposure to ultraviolet rays and may result in first- and second-degree burns. Deeper burns may result from careless use of sunlamps. Although sunburn rarely requires hospitalization, it may be incapacitating for several days because of pain, swelling, and such systemic effects as fever and headache. The time between exposure and the development of symptoms is usually from 4 to 12 hours.

First aid for sunburn is the same as for first- and second-degree burns. If later medical treatment appears likely, do not apply ointment to the sunburn. Any person with extensive sunburn (10 percent or more of the body surface in a child and 15 percent or more in an adult) should be seen by a physician. Likewise, very deep burns with many large blisters should have medical treatment. If blisters break, apply a dry, sterile dressing.

10

EXPOSURE TO RADIATION

Nuclear weapon detonations are characterized by the release of tremendous amounts of heat and energy and by immediate and delayed radiation effects, including fallout. Distance from the explosion, protection afforded by nearby buildings, and duration of exposure will determine the extent of exposure to radioactivity.

Instructions on survival from radioactive fallout have been prepared by civil defense agencies and other groups concerned with preparedness for disaster. The most important principles are: (1) that radioactive fallout "decays" (loses its potency) with time, (2) that radioactive dust can be washed off the hair, the body, and food containers with soap and water, and (3) that proper shelter will greatly increase the chances of survival.

Emergency handling of cases of exposure to radiation or to radioactive substances demands little more than common sense.

Giving first aid treatment in cases where a victim has been exposed to external radiation or internal radiation by ingestion or inhalation of radioactive substances normally presents little hazard to the first-aider.

In cases that involve external contamination of the body or clothing by radioactive materials, such as liquids or dirt, and that may be complicated by injuries, especially wounds, some practical steps should be taken to confine contamination:

- Wear disposable gloves and other clothing.
- Wrap the victim in blankets.
- Care for the victim's injuries.
- Get the victim to appropriate facilities for decontamination.

Whether injuries exist or not, get the victim to adequate medical facilities, preferably an authorized center for care of radiation accidents. The facility should be notified in advance that a person exposed to radiation is being taken there.

Get personnel trained in radiation hazards to the site where the injury occurred for the purpose of radiation survey. The first-aider, the victim, and all clothing and equipment must be monitored and decontaminated as necessary.

11

COLD EXPOSURE AND FROSTBITE

The extent of injury caused by exposure to abnormally low temperature generally depends on such factors as wind velocity, type and duration of exposure, temperature, and humidity.

Freezing is accelerated by wind, humidity, or a combination of the two. Injury caused by cold, dry air will be less than that caused by cold, moist air or exposure to cold air while wearing wet clothing. Fatigue, smoking, drinking of alcoholic beverages, emotional stress, and the presence of wounds or fractures intensify the harmful effects of cold.

SIGNS AND SYMPTOMS

The general manifestations of prolonged exposure to extreme cold include shivering, numbness, low body temperature, drowsiness, and marked muscular weakness. As time passes, there is mental confusion and impairment of judgment. The victim staggers, his eyesight fails, he falls, and he may become unconscious. Shock is evident, and the victim's heart may develop fibrillation. Death, if it occurs, is usually due to heart failure.

Frostbite results when crystals form, either superficially or deeply in the fluids and the underlying soft tissues of the skin. The effects are more severe if the injured area is thawed and then refrozen. Frostbite is the most common injury caused by exposure to the cold elements. Usually, the frozen area is small. The nose, cheeks, ears, fingers, and toes are most commonly affected.

Just before frostbite occurs, the affected skin may be slightly flushed. The skin changes to white or grayish yellow as the frostbite develops (Fig. 86). Pain is sometimes felt early but subsides later. Often, there is no pain; the part feels intensely cold and numb. The victim commonly is not aware of frostbite until someone tells him or

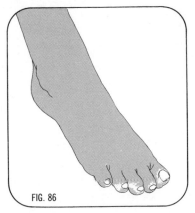

FIG. 86

until he observes his pale, glossy skin. The extent of local injury cannot be determined accurately on initial examination, even after rewarming. The extent of tissue damage usually corresponds to that in burns. In superficial frostbite, there will be an area that looks white or grayish, and the surface skin will feel hard, but the underlying tissue will be soft. With deeper involvement, large blisters appear on the surface, as well as in underlying tissue, and the affected area is hard, cold, and insensitive. Destruction of the entire thickness of the skin will necessitate skin grafting. If freezing is deeper than the skin, tissue destruction will be severe and will constitute a medical emergency, because gangrene may result from loss of blood supply to the injured part.

FIRST AID

The objectives of first aid are to protect the frozen area from further injury, to warm the affected area rapidly, and to maintain respiration. Formerly, it was recommended that victims of frostbite be treated by slow warming—rubbing with snow and gradually increasing the temperature. But recent studies have shown conclusively that much better results are obtained if the affected part is *warmed rapidly* in running or circulating water, unless the part has been thawed and refrozen, in which case it should be warmed at room temperature (from 70° F to 74° F). Do not use excessive heat, as from a stove, hot water bottles, electric blankets, or other devices.

Frostbite

• Cover the frozen part.
• Provide extra clothing and blankets.

- Bring the victim indoors as soon as possible.
- Give him a warm drink.
- Rewarm the frozen part *quickly* by immersing it in water that is warm but not hot. Test the water by pouring some over the inner surface of your forearm or place a thermometer in the water and carefully add warm water to keep the temperature between 102° F and 105° F (Fig. 87). If warm water is not available or practical to use, wrap the affected part gently in a sheet and warm blankets.

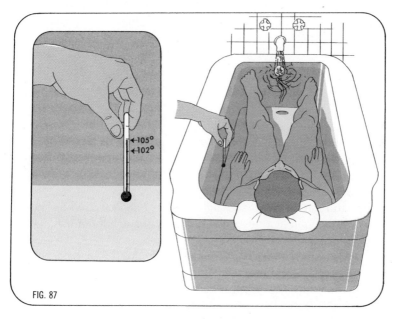

FIG. 87

- Handle the area of frostbite *gently* and *do not massage it.* Severe swelling will develop very rapidly after thawing. Discontinue warming as soon as the part becomes flushed. Once the part is rewarmed, have the victim exercise it.
- Cleanse the affected area with water and either soap or a mild detergent (not laundry or dishwasher detergent). Rinse it thoroughly. Carefully blot it dry with sterile or clean towels. Do not break blisters.
- If the victim's fingers or toes are involved, place dry, sterile gauze between them to keep them separated.
- Do not apply other dressings unless the victim is to be transported to medical aid.
- Elevate frostbitten parts and protect them from contact with bedclothes.

- Do not allow the victim to walk after the affected part thaws, if his feet are involved.
- Do not apply additional heat and do not allow the victim to sit near a radiator, stove, or fire. (NOTE. If a person with frozen feet is alone and must walk to get medical assistance, he should not attempt thawing in advance.)
- If travel after receiving first aid is necessary, cover the affected parts with a sterile or clean cloth.
- Obtain medical assistance as soon as possible. If the distance to be covered is great, apply temporary dressings to affected hands.
- Keep injured parts elevated during transportation.
- Give fluids as described in chapter 9 provided that the victim is conscious and not vomiting.

Prolonged Exposure

- Give the victim artificial respiration, if necessary.
- Bring the victim into a warm room as quickly as possible.
- Remove wet or frozen clothing and anything that constricts the victim's arms, legs, or fingers and might interfere with circulation as the frozen part is thawed and swelling begins.
- Rewarm the victim rapidly by wrapping him in warm blankets or by placing him in a tub of water that is warm, but not hot to your hand and forearm.
- If the victim is conscious, give him hot liquids (but not alcohol) by mouth.
- Dry the victim thoroughly if water was used to rewarm him.
- Carry out appropriate procedures as described under frostbite.

12

HEAT STROKE, HEAT CRAMPS, AND HEAT EXHAUSTION

Excessive heat may affect the body in a variety of ways, which result in several conditions referred to as heat stroke, heat cramps, and heat exhaustion.

DEFINITIONS

Heat stroke is a response to heat characterized by extremely high body temperature and disturbance of the sweating mechanism.

Heat cramps are musuclar pains and spasms due largely to loss of salt from the body in sweating or to inadequate intake of salt. The cramps are more severe if the victim has drunk a large quantity of tap water or soft drinks without replacing the salt deficiency, in which case severe mental confusion and even convulsions may develop. Heat cramps may be associated with heat exhaustion.

Heat exhaustion is a response to heat characterized by fatigue, weakness, and collapse due to inadequate intake of water to compensate for loss of fluids through sweating.

CAUSES

Heat reactions are brought about by both internal and external factors. The extent of overheating is determined by the relation of the temperature of the environment to—

- The temperature of the body.
- The amount of air circulating around the body.
- The amount of moisture in the environment (the humidity).
- The kind and amount of clothing worn.

Ordinarily, body temperature is kept stable by conduction of heat through the body and radiation of heat from the body surface, by movement of air around the body, and by evaporation of sweat. Harmful effects occur when the body becomes overheated and cannot eliminate the excess heat, or when large amounts of water or salt or both are lost through profuse sweating after strenuous exercise or manual labor in an extremely hot atmosphere.

Elderly persons, small children, chronic invalids, alcoholics, and overweight persons are particularly susceptible to heat reactions, especially during heat waves in areas where a moderate climate usually prevails.

SIGNS, SYMPTOMS, AND FIRST AID

Heat Stroke

In heat stroke, the body temperature may be 106° F or higher. The victim's skin is characteristically hot, red, and dry (Fig. 88). (The sweating mechanism is blocked.) The pulse is rapid and strong, and the victim may be unconscious. Heat stroke is an immediate life-threatening problem. Because the mortality rate associated with heat stroke is high, *first aid* should be directed toward *immediate* measures to cool the body quickly. Take care, however, to prevent overchilling of the victim once his temperature goes below 102° F. The following first aid measures are applicable whenever a person's body temperature reaches 105° F:

- Undress the victim and, using a small bath towel to maintain modesty, repeatedly sponge his bare skin with cool water or rubbing alcohol; *or* apply cold packs continuously; *or* place him in a tub of cold water (do not add ice) until his temperature is sufficiently lowered, and then dry him off.
- Use fans or air conditioners, if available, because drafts will promote cooling.
- If the victim's temperature starts to go up again, start the cooling process again.
- Do not give the victim stimulants.

Heat Cramps

Heat cramps are often an early sign of approaching heat exhaustion, if there is a deficiency in both water and salt. The muscles of

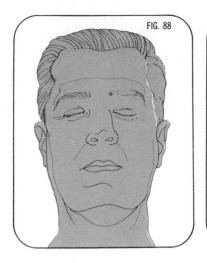

FIG. 88

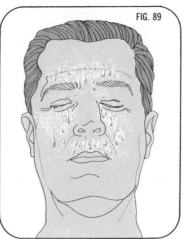

FIG. 89

the victim's legs and abdomen are likely to be affected first. *First aid* measures include the following:

- Give the victim sips of salt water (1 teaspoonful of salt per glass), half a glass every 15 minutes, over a period of about 1 hour.
- Exert pressure with your hands on the cramped muscles, or gently massage them, to help relieve spasm.

Heat Exhaustion

In heat exhaustion, the body temperature is normal, or nearly normal. There is excessive pooling of blood in the capillaries of the skin, in the body's effort to lose heat. This pooling interferes with the circulation to vital organs, such as the brain, heart, and lungs. As the body tries to compensate for the reduced supply of blood to critical areas, the smaller veins constrict, and the skin becomes white or pale and cool and clammy (Fig. 89). The victim may faint but will probably regain consciousness as his head is lowered and the blood supply to his brain is improved. The victim complains of great weakness, nausea and dizziness, and perhaps cramps. *First aid* measures include the following:

- Give the victim sips of salt water (1 teaspoonful of salt per glass), half a glass every 15 minutes, over a period of about 1 hour.
- Have the victim lie down; raise his feet from 8 to 12 inches.
- Loosen his clothing.

- Apply cool, wet cloths and fan the victim, or move him to an air-conditioned room.
- If the victim vomits, do not give him any more fluids. Take him as soon as possible to a hospital, where intravenous salt solution can be given.
- After an attack of heat exhaustion, the victim should be advised not to return to work for several days and should be protected from exposure to abnormally warm temperature.

13

BONE AND JOINT INJURIES

DEFINITIONS

Multiple injuries to the skeletal system—including the bones, joints, and ligaments—and to the adjacent soft tissues are common in all types of major accidents. A break or a crack in a bone is called a *fracture*. A *dislocation* is an injury to the capsule and ligaments of a joint that results in displacement of a bone end at a joint. The association of a dislocation with a fracture is called a *fracture dislocation*. A *sprain* is an injury to a joint ligament or a muscle tendon in the region of a joint; it involves the partial tearing or stretching of these structures, injuries to blood vessels, and contusions of the surrounding soft tissue without dislocation or fracture. A *strain* is an injury to a muscle that results from overstretching; it may be associated with a sprain or a fracture.

FRACTURES

Classification

Closed (or *simple*) fractures are those not related to open wounds on the surface of the body, although there may be a laceration over or near a fracture site (Fig. 90).

Open (or *compound*) fractures are those associated directly with open wounds (Fig. 91). An open fracture may result from external violence or may be produced by injury from within, as broken ends of a bone protrude through the skin at the time of the accident or later through motion or mishandling of the fractured bone. In an open fracture, the wound usually is inflicted by a broken bone end

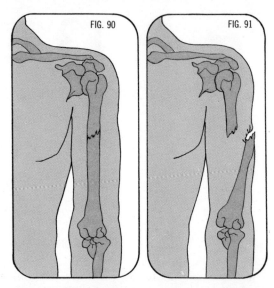

that tears through the skin and slips back again. Sometimes the cause is a missile, such as a bullet, that penetrates the skin and breaks a bone. Open fractures are much more serious than closed ones, because the fracture area is always contaminated, and infection is virtually certain unless prevented by prompt, effective treatment.

Causes

The most common causes of fractures are motor vehicle accidents, falls, and accidents related to recreational sports and activities. Some fractures result from very slight injuries, particularly in older people, because of brittle or abnormal bones.

Motor vehicle accidents are responsible for more than 50,000 deaths each year and for over 1.5 million disabling injuries. Nearly half the fatalities occur on weekends; and, although there are approximately the same number of deaths during the day as at night, the death *rate* in automobile accidents is higher in the late afternoon and early evening hours than at any other time of the day. The highest accident rate is reported among drivers between the ages of 15 and 24. Over twice as many deaths occur in rural areas as in towns and cities, where almost half the victims are pedestrians. In automobile accidents, the condition of the vehicle (such as defects in lights, turn indicators, brakes, exhaust system, and tires) is responsible for only a small percentage of casualties, although it may be a contributing factor in many more. Speeding, other improper driving practices (such as failure to yield the right of way, driving to the left of the center line, and tailgating) and the condition of the driver cause most of the accidents. Drowsiness, falling asleep, fatigue, inattention, alcoholic beverages, medications, and emotional factors are responsible for many serious injuries and deaths each year.

Falls are responsible for almost 20,000 deaths a year. Three-fourths of all falls are experienced by elderly persons, and three-fourths occur in the home environment.

Signs and Symptoms

If an accident victim is conscious, he will usually be able to provide clues to possible fractures. He may recall his position before the injury and relate what happened as he fell or struck some object. He may have heard or felt a bone snap and be able to indicate the location of pain or tenderness or may have difficulty in moving an injured part. He may also report a grating sensation of broken bones rubbing together (called crepitus) and abnormal motion in some area of his body.

Other signs of fracture include—
• Differences in the shape and length of corresponding bones on the two sides of the victim's body.
• Obvious deformities, such as angulation, crookedness, shortening or rotation of a limb, or an open wound over a bone.
• Swelling (which may not be evident at first but develops rapidly) and discoloration of the overlying skin due to hemorrhage.
• Pain or tenderness in response to gentle pressure at the site of a suspected fracture.

Closed fractures are much more common than open fractures. As a rule, accurate diagnosis can be made only by a physician with the assistance of X-ray examination, but the first-aider should *suspect* that a bone is broken when any of the signs are present. Even if there is doubt, to prevent aggravation of existing injuries, he should carry out first aid measures for a fracture.

First Aid Principles

The first aid objectives in fractures are to provide all necessary first aid care, to keep the broken bone ends and adjacent joints from moving, and to give care for shock. Steps are—
• Provide first aid for airway obstruction. Restore respiration. Give first aid for severe bleeding, pain, shock, and other emergencies.

- After rescue, if it is necessary, protect against further injury. Call for an ambulance, if it is warranted, or medical assistance.
- Prevent motion of the injured parts and the adjacent joints. Elevate involved limbs, if possible, without disturbing suspected fractures.
- Apply splints if modern ambulance service is not available, if there is a delay in transportation, or in less serious injuries before seeking medical assistance for diagnosis and treatment.

The first-aider should not attempt to set (or reduce) a fracture that requires restoration of bone fragments to normal position and correct alignment and should never attempt to straighten a deformity that involves a joint.

If an ambulance or rescue squad can arrive within a short period after an accident, when an injured person obviously requires hospitalization, do not attempt to move the victim unless there is danger of fire, carbon monoxide poisoning, explosion, drowning, or other life-threatening emergency. Above all, in attempting rescue, do not drag victims out of vehicles or from under wreckage or throw them on the ground in your haste to save their lives. If possible, even in the midst of a crowded street or highway, take the time to tie a victim's injured leg to his uninjured one or bind his injured arm to his chest or side. Lift and move an unconscious victim as though there is injury to his neck or spine. Wait for adequate help—at least three and preferably four persons—and obtain a rigid support for the victim's back, if possible. After an injury during water sports, float the victim to shore without bending his neck or back. *Do not* lift the victim out of the water without a back support. Delegate others to telephone for an ambulance and the police, if necessary, and to assist in maintaining order in the area of the accident.

If an *open fracture* is evident or suspected, treat the wound as outlined previously. Remove or cut away the victim's clothing and control hemorrhage by applying pressure through a large sterile (or clean) dressing over the wound. Do not wash the wound, do not probe it, and do not insert your fingers into it.

If a fragment of bone is protruding, cover the entire wound with a large, sterile bandage compress or pads; if these are not available, use freshly laundered sheets or towels. Do *not* replace the bone fragment, because it will carry foreign material and harmful bacteria deep into the wound, increasing the danger of infection.

Apply splints, as described below, according to the location of the fracture. Then elevate the limb slightly to reduce hemorrhage and swelling. Open fractures should have priority over closed fractures for transportation and medical treatment, unless associated injuries dictate otherwise.

The following illustrations will provide reference charts for the primary bones (Fig. 92) and muscles (Fig. 93) in the body.

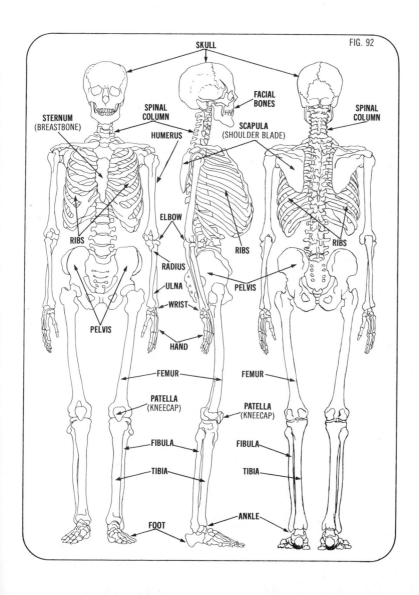

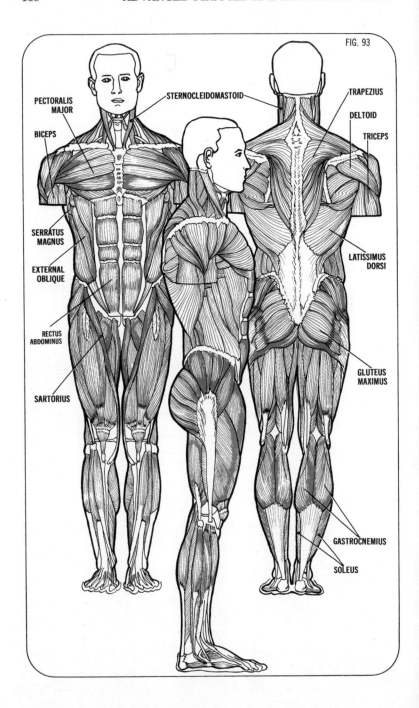

FIG. 93

Splinting

Splints are devices applied to arms, legs, or trunk to immobilize an injured part when a fracture is suspected. They decrease pain and the likelihood of shock by preventing motion of broken bone ends and adjacent joints. They also protect against further injury during transportation for medical treatment.

Splints are of two main types: fixation and traction. *Fixation splints* are applied to immobilize broken ends of a bone and adjacent joints. *Traction splints* may be used on long bones of the legs to relieve muscle spasm and to prevent overriding of the fractured bone ends.

Many types of splints are available commercially; however, the first aid worker's access to any of these is unlikely, unless he becomes a member of an ambulance team or works in an industrial clinic. Therefore, learn to make and apply improvised splints. A simple splinting technique in an emergency is to tape or tie an injured leg to the uninjured one—with padding between, if possible (Fig. 94)—or to bind an injured arm, after padding, to the victim's chest if the elbow is bent or to the side if the elbow is straight.

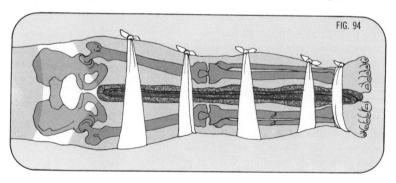

FIG. 94

A pillow may be used as a splint if it can be tied or pinned around a fracture in an accessible location, such as a knee or foot. Satisfactory emergency splints can be constructed from corrugated cardboard cartons. Bend the cardboard along longitudinal creases to form a three-sided box (Fig. 95) to support a fracture of an upper arm, forearm, or lower leg and ankle, or the entire leg of a child, provided that hemorrhage is not a problem and that adequate padding can be procured for protection of the limb from the stiff, rough edges of the cardboard. Boards, sticks, and rolled-up blankets or newspapers can be used as splints. They should be long enough to extend past the joints on either side of a suspected fracture. It may

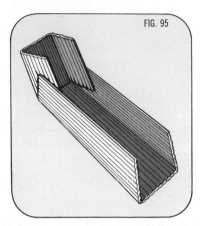

FIG. 95

be necessary to tie two splints together to give the necessary length. Place adequate padding or cloth, clothing, pillows, paper, or other bulky material between the splint and the victim's skin, especially over bony prominences, and wrap the ends of board splints well, unless they extend beyond the body.

Use handkerchiefs, cravat bandages (see Figs. 158A through 158D page 207), neckties, belts, or strips of torn cloth to tie splints in place. Joints should be immobilized above and below the location of the suspected fracture. In fractures of an arm, check the pulse in the wrist and inspect the fingers often for swelling, bluish discoloration, or marked pallor of the skin, which may result if the bandages are too tight. If the victim complains of numbness, tingling sensations, or inability to move his fingers or toes, loosen ties immediately— otherwise permanent nerve damage may result. If splints are used in fractures of legs or feet and these symptoms appear, loosen the bandages, remove the victim's shoes and hose, and examine his toes repeatedly for color changes or swelling. If these signs appear, it may be necessary to further loosen bandages and reapply them.

FIRST AID FOR SPECIFIC FRACTURES

Skull (Fig. 96)

The skull consists of 8 bones that form the cranium (which encloses the brain) and 14 facial bones. Only the lower jaw is movable.

In infancy, the bones of the cranium are separated by membrane in six areas; these spaces (the fontanelles) can be identified as soft spots, which disappear as the bones fuse. The largest fontanelle, in the frontal region, normally closes within from 12 to 18 months after

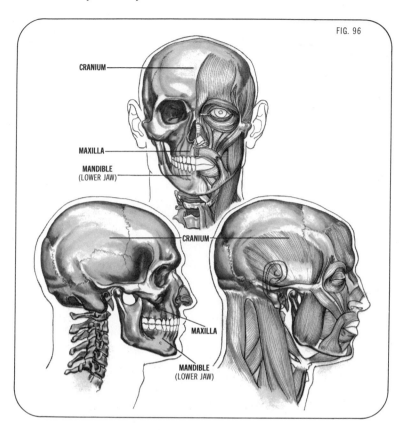

FIG. 96

CRANIUM

MAXILLA

MANDIBLE
(LOWER JAW)

CRANIUM

MAXILLA

MANDIBLE
(LOWER JAW)

birth; the others normally close within 12 months. Pulsation in the large fontanelle can be seen in an infant who has little covering hair. Slight swelling or bulging in the area is not normal, except when the infant is crying or straining, and may represent either an accumulation of cerebrospinal fluid or swelling of the brain due to injury. In an adult, the bones are fused or tightly joined by connective tissue.

The term "skull fracture" usually refers to a fracture of the cranium. This injury is important chiefly because it may be associated with brain damage. Wounds of the brain may be produced by displaced fragments of bone; pressure injury to brain tissue may occur as the result of a depressed fracture without an overlying wound. The most serious skull fractures include those produced by severe falls with crushing injury and those produced by external objects such as bullets and flying particles of glass and metal, which can drive hair, scalp, bone particles, and dirt into the brain. Drainage of cerebrospinal fluid from the victim's ears and nose in cases of skull fracture is discussed in chapter 3, as are wounds of the scalp and first aid for brain injury. Remember that an unconscious victim of a skull fracture may also have a fracture of the spine.

Face

Fractures of the facial bones are suggested by distortion of the victim's features, numbness, pain, severe bruising and swelling, bleeding from the victim's nose and mouth, limited motion of his jaw, and failure of his teeth to meet normally.

Double vision may indicate that the bone around the victim's eye is fractured. Often in the early period after injury, before severe swelling has developed, fractures may be detected by feeling irregularities in the bones of the victim's face.

Fractures of the face may be associated with blunt injury or with severe wounds, in which case control of hemorrhage and establishment of an open airway are of immediate importance. If the victim is conscious and has no evidence of neck or back injury, prop him up and have him lean forward so that blood and other secretions can drain out. If he is unconscious, turn him on his side or abdomen to permit drainage. With either the conscious or unconscious victim, if a *neck injury* is not suspected, and there is evidence of airway obstruction, tilt the victim's head back and arch his neck; support his head with your hand or a small cloth pad; and pull the jaw fragments up or hold his tongue down or forward. If a neck injury is suspected, do not tilt his head but pull his tongue forward if necessary to prevent airway obstruction.

If a rubber bulb of any kind is available, suck out blood and other secretions from the back of the victim's throat. Place a loose bandage beneath his chin, tied in a bow at the top of his head to hold face dressings in place or to relieve displacement of his chin downward, but *never* apply a bandage in such a way that the victim cannot open his mouth to vomit or to permit drainage of blood.

Spine and Vertebrae (Fig. 97)

The backbone, or spinal column, is composed of 33 bones called vertebrae. There are 7 in the neck, 12 in the chest region, and 5 in the lumbar region. The sacrum consists of 5 fused vertebrae and forms a part of the pelvis. The remaining 4 form the tailbone, or coccyx. The upper 24 vertebrae are separated by plates or disks of cartilage. Occasionally, because of a blow, twisting, or heavy lifting, a disk may slip out of place. The backbone encases the spinal cord,

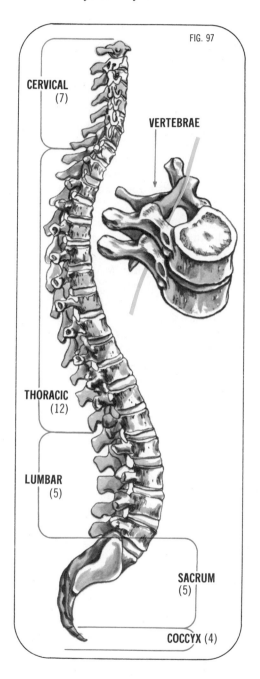

FIG. 97

CERVICAL
(7)

VERTEBRAE

THORACIC
(12)

LUMBAR
(5)

SACRUM
(5)

COCCYX (4)

which passes through circular openings in the separate vertebrae. If a vertebra or disk is fractured or dislocated, the spinal cord may be injured, and loss of motion and sensation below the level of injury may result.

The spine in the *neck* region can be fractured and dislocated at the same time by a severe blow to the head, which may occur in an automobile or diving accident or be caused by a falling object. The victim usually has severe pain, spasm of his neck muscles, and difficulty in moving his head. If the spinal cord has been injured only slightly, there will be weakness and numbness below the level of injury. More serious damage will cause paralysis and loss of sensation.

A victim's inability to move his arms and legs after an accident must always be considered to be due to injury of the spinal cord if the limbs themselves are uninjured.

Fractures of the neck vertebrae without injury to the spinal cord respond well to treatment. It is very important for the first aid worker not to allow the victim's head to be bent forward or backward or to be moved from side to side. If the victim is having breathing difficulty, rescuers must follow the steps of airway control, the only modification being that head tilt should be minimal and forward displacement of the mandible and positive pressure breathing should be accomplished first if indicated. Seek medical advice and send for an ambulance with trained personnel to assist in moving the victim.

If you must move a person with a suspected fracture of the neck vertebrae, place him on his back for transportation. But do not move him without the help of at least three (preferably four) persons—all of whom clearly understand the best method of keeping the victim's head and trunk as rigid as possible, without twisting, bending, or side-to-side motion—while slipping a solid board, a door, or a shutter underneath to support the entire back. If helpers have not been previously trained, it is best to practice briefly on an uninjured person at the scene of the accident before attempting to move the victim. With the victim lying on his back, a small pad or towel may be placed in the space under his neck (Fig. 98). (Do not put a pillow under his head.) Then place rolled-up clothing, blankets, or sandbags around his head, neck, and shoulders to prevent motion (Fig. 99). Anchor the restraining materials with bricks or stones, if these are available. One person should steady the victim's head by placing his palms at the sides of the victim's head, spreading out his fingers, and extending them down onto the victim's shoulders so that the victim's

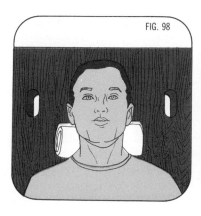

FIG. 98

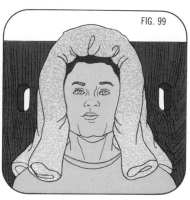

FIG. 99

head and neck are splinted and supported as they lie in the cradle of the helper's hands. The victim's neck should be kept in a straight line with the center of his trunk. Secure the victim to the backboard with several bandages or improvised ties (Figs. 100 and 101).

In water accidents that happen during swimming, diving, surfing, or boating, in which the victim's neck appears to be injured, keep

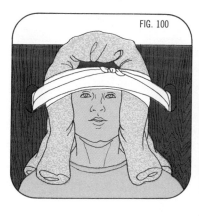

FIG. 100

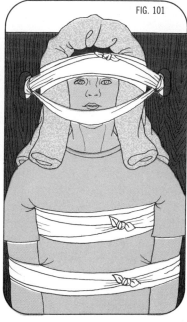

FIG. 101

the victim floating by placing one of your hands under his shoulders and head. Keep his head immobile until a board, stretcher, or other rigid support can be obtained. He must be lifted carefully from the water onto a dock or a boat while he is on the support (see chapter 6). An open airway and respiration must be maintained.

Trunk Region (Fig. 102)

Fractures of the upper and lower back regions of the spine are common in motor vehicle accidents, especially when a passenger is thrown out of the vehicle or has his spine bent acutely forward at the time of injury, so that the body of the vertebra is fractured by compression.

A fracture of the spine should be suspected if the victim has pain at the affected site and extending around his chest or abdomen or down his legs, along the course of his spinal nerves, as well as

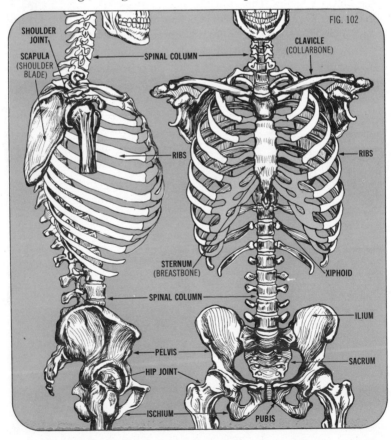

FIG. 102

SHOULDER JOINT
SCAPULA (SHOULDER BLADE)
SPINAL COLUMN
CLAVICLE (COLLARBONE)
RIBS
RIBS
STERNUM (BREASTBONE)
XIPHOID
SPINAL COLUMN
ILIUM
PELVIS
SACRUM
HIP JOINT
ISCHIUM
PUBIS

tenderness over the area of injury, and muscle spasm. If the spinal cord is affected, there will be weakness or paralysis and disturbance of sensation below the level of injury.

Handle the victim of a suspected spine fracture as little as possible. Send for an ambulance. Until help arrives, leave the victim in the position in which he was found, unless there is delay in transportation or his condition is critical. Take care of other emergencies, such as difficulty in breathing, hemorrhage, and open wounds, and apply dressings and splints as necessary. If the victim must be moved, obtain a door, a long, wide board, or other rigid material to support his back. With three or four helpers, roll the victim part way onto his side, holding his head in a straight line with his trunk; slip the board as far under his body as possible from behind; then slide him over onto the board (see Figs. 242 through 246, page 280). Do not twist his neck or back. Arrange rolled-up blankets or clothing on both sides of his trunk, head, and neck for immobilization. Anchor the victim securely to the board and handle him gently.

Accident victims with back injury may also be lifted as described above for neck injuries. As an emergency measure, a person with a suspected back injury who is in a position of grave danger and must be rescued immediately may be carefully rolled face down onto a blanket for transportation to safety (see chapter 17). Never allow such a victim, however, to stand, walk, or sit up if a fracture of his spine is likely.

Pelvis (Fig. 103)

The pelvis is a girdle of fused bones that forms the floor of the trunk. The sacrum in the back, which is made up of five vertebrae, joins with the pelvic bone or hipbone on each side. Each pelvic bone is actually made up of three bones, the ilium, the ischium, and the pubis. The head of the femur (the thighbone) fits into a socket in the pelvic bone, and the two pelvic bones join in front in the pubic region. The pelvic cavity contains the urethra, the bladder, the lower part of the bowel, and, in the female, the uterus and the vagina. Any of these structures may be injured when the pelvis is fractured, and severe internal bleeding may result if large blood vessels are torn by a fragment of bone. Pelvic fractures, rather common in automobile accidents, produce marked pain at the point of fracture. If the internal organs are injured, the victim usually develops severe shock and a paralysis of the bowel.

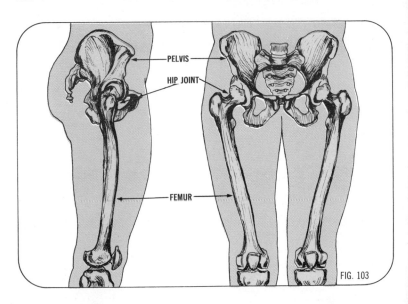

PELVIS

HIP JOINT

FEMUR

FIG. 103

Pelvic injuries are extremely serious, and *first aid* should be the same as for suspected fractures of the spine: Handle the victim as little as possible; obtain a firm, wide, rigid support for his back if a stretcher is not available; and keep him on his back during transportation. If neither thigh appears to be fractured, the victim's knees may be bent and a pillow may be placed underneath to reduce abdominal pain.

Ribs and Sternum (Fig. 104)

There are 12 ribs connected to each side of the spinal column in the chest region. Ten of these are joined to the sternum (or breastbone) in front by cartilage; the other two, the lowest, are very short and are called floating ribs. From the upper end of the sternum, the clavicle (collarbone), a long, thin bone, passes horizontally to join the scapula (shoulder blade) near the tip of the shoulder. These bones, with the spinal column in this region, make up the rib cage, which protects the heart, lungs, and other structures in the chest and assists, through movement of the muscles of the chest wall, in breathing. Fractures of a single rib and small cracks in several ribs (often due to a direct blow or fall) produce pain and discomfort but, as a rule, are not otherwise serious.

In crushing wounds of the chest, in which several ribs are fractured, perhaps in several places each, breathing is greatly impaired,

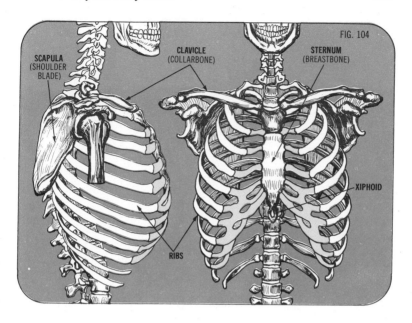

and the victim's life may be endangered. In addition, the lungs may be punctured as a rib is displaced from its normal position, allowing air, and perhaps blood, to escape into the chest cavity. This accumulation of air and blood between the lung and the chest wall may compress lung tissue. Often, if a person's lung has been punctured, he will cough up bright red blood. If a fractured rib has been driven down into the liver or spleen, severe internal bleeding and shock will develop.

As first aid for rib fractures without other injury, place an elastic bandage or several flat, broad cravat bandages (see page 207). Figs. 158A through 158D) around the lower half of the victim's chest to restrict chest movements and give some relief of pain (Fig. 105). Make certain, however, that there is no interference with breathing. A sucking wound of the chest produced by a puncture wound or a compound fracture of the ribs is a major emergency. It requires immediate closure by strapping a large pad or plastic or metal foil over the wound until a dressing is available; the first aid worker may seal the opening with his hand. In crushing injuries of the chest in which stability of the chest wall is lost, so that the lung cannot expand on the affected side, some benefit may be obtained by placing a circular dressing around the injured area and turning the victim onto his back without pressing on any part of his chest. Send

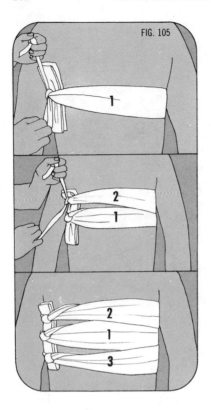

FIG. 105

for medical aid, or transport the victim to a hospital in an ambulance. Prop the victim's head up. Watch for signs of acute distress in breathing. Keep the victim's airway open. Oxygen should be provided as soon as available.

Fractures of the sternum, which are rare, are produced by severe, external force, as when a person is thrown forward against a steering wheel or dashboard in an automobile crash. First aid is the same as for multiple rib fractures.

Clavicle (Fig. 106)

Fractures of the clavicle, or collarbone, usually occur in the weakest portion, which is one-third of the distance from the tip of the shoulder to the sternum. These fractures are particularly common in children and ordinarily heal without complication in 2 or 3 weeks (twice as long in adults). First aid consists of applying a sling to elevate the victim's arm and shoulder blade, which fall because of the loss of support from the clavicle, and then binding the arm to the victim's chest.

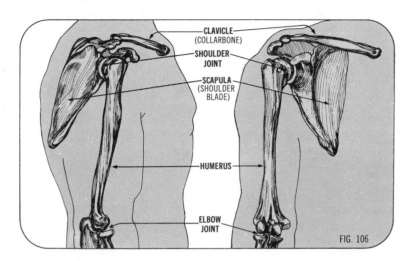

CLAVICLE (COLLARBONE)
SHOULDER JOINT
SCAPULA (SHOULDER BLADE)
HUMERUS
ELBOW JOINT
FIG. 106

Prepare a triangular piece of cloth approximately 55 inches across the base and from 36 to 40 inches along the sides. Regular triangular bandages of this size may also be purchased in unit packages.

Place one end of the bandage on the uninjured side and let the other end hang down in front of the chest, parallel to the side of the body. Carry the point behind the elbow of the injured arm (Fig. 107A). Carry the second end of the bandage up over the shoulder (Fig. 107B) and tie the two ends together at the side of the neck (not over the spine). Bring the point of the bandage forward and pin it to the front of the sling. If a pin is not available, twist the point of the

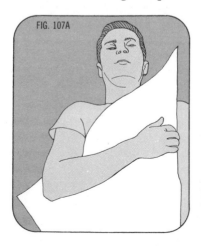

FIG. 107A

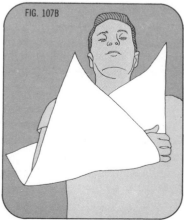

FIG. 107B

bandage until it is snug at the elbow (Fig. 107C) and tie a single knot (Fig. 107D). The ends of the fingers should extend just beyond the base so that the first-aider can observe whether or not the circulation is cut off. Using a thin board if available, slide a wide cravat under the victim at the small of his back (Fig. 107E). Slide the cravat up to his chest and complete by tying snugly on the uninjured side (Fig. 107F). (Also see Fig. 108.) The victim should be seen by a physician soon after injury.

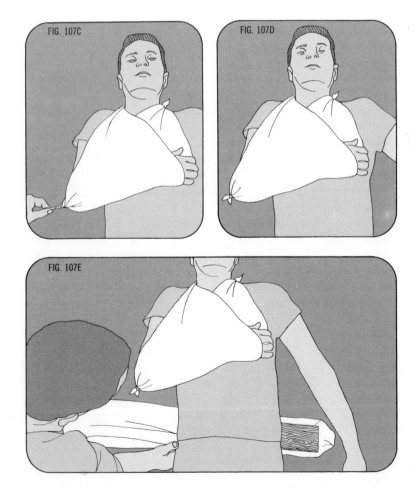

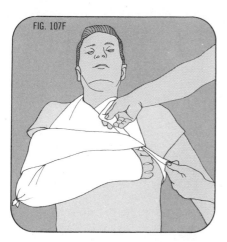

FIG. 107F

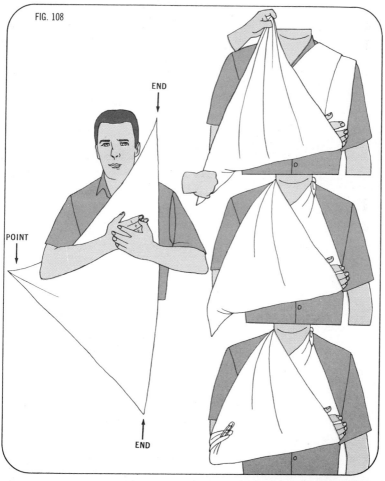

FIG. 108

END

POINT

END

Shoulder and Upper Arm

A fracture of the scapula (shoulder blade) is generally the direct result of the impact of a fall or an automobile collision; dislocations of the shoulder joint, sprains, and contusions are common in this area. First aid consists of applying a sling and bandaging the victim's upper arm to his chest wall (Figs. 109 and 110).

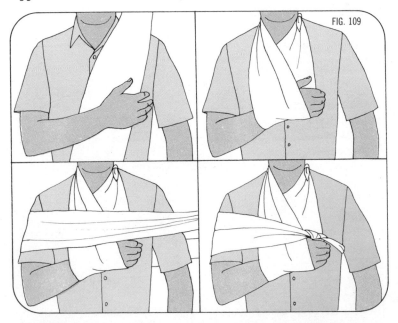

FIG. 109

Fracture of the humerus, the bone in the upper arm, may be overlooked if the break is close to the shoulder, because the fracture may be impacted and cause less disability than if the injury were in the shaft of the bone, where false motion may be present and the pain may be more acute.

For a closed fracture of the humerus, place a pad in the victim's armpit. Apply a splint or improvised splint, tied in place above and below the break area (Fig. 111). Support the forearm with a sling that does not produce upward pressure at the fracture site (Fig. 112). Bind the victim's upper arm to his chest wall (Fig. 113). For an open fracture, cover the wound with a large sterile or clean dressing and apply a splint that does not press against the area of the break. Do not attempt to cleanse the wound. In the absence of a splint, support the victim's arm with a sling and bind it to his chest with an encircling bandage.

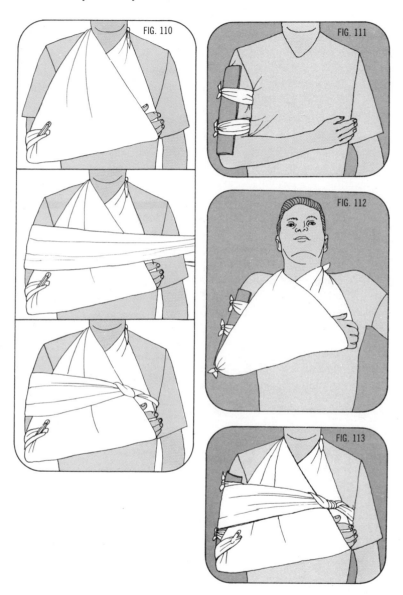

FIG. 110
FIG. 111
FIG. 112
FIG. 113

Elbow (Fig. 114)

Elbow fractures may involve the lower part of the humerus or the bones of the forearm. If the victim's elbow was bent at the time of injury, do not try to straighten it. Place his forearm in a sling and bind it to his body. If the fracture occurred with the elbow straight, do not attempt to bend it to apply a sling. After placing a protective fold of cloth in the victim's armpit, secure a well-padded splint with ties along both sides of the elbow. Have the victim lie down and elevate his arm. If a splint is not available, wrap a pillow about the arm, centering it at the elbow, and tie or pin the two sides together.

In all fractures of the arm, elbow, or forearm, there is great danger of damage to the nerves and blood vessels that supply the hand. Such damage may be produced by direct injury from splintered bone, but all too often it is the result of constriction from bandages used to hold dressings or splints in place. Ordinarily, it takes time for swelling of the tissues to develop, but it may be necessary to loosen ties—even if they were correctly applied—immediately after injury. Keep the victim's hand raised and inspect his fingers often. Check the pulse at the wrist. If the pulse cannot be felt, if there is marked swelling, or if the victim complains of throbbing and numbness in his hand, loosen the ties and reapply them. Tight bandages or hemorrhage may cause a bluish discoloration of the victim's fingers. Extreme pallor of the hand usually means that no circulation can reach the area.

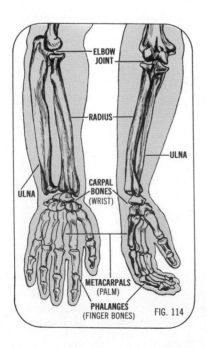

ELBOW JOINT

RADIUS

ULNA

ULNA

CARPAL BONES (WRIST)

METACARPALS (PALM)

PHALANGES (FINGER BONES)   FIG. 114

Forearm and Wrist (Fig. 114)

The two bones of the forearm may be fractured individually or together. The ulna, the inner bone when the arm is held out with the palm up, forms a hinge joint with the humerus at the elbow; it narrows considerably at the wrist. The radius, the other bone in the forearm, extends the length of the forearm, is widest at the hand end, and supports the hand. It rotates in an arc about the ulna as the hand and forearm are turned palm up or palm down. Fractures in the midportion of the forearm are treated in the same way as fractures of the shaft of the humerus: Apply well-padded splints on each side—or use a padded, improvised splint—such as a magazine (Figs. 115 and 116); bend the victim's elbow; and apply a sling,

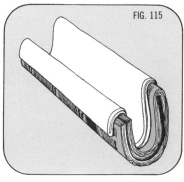

FIG. 115

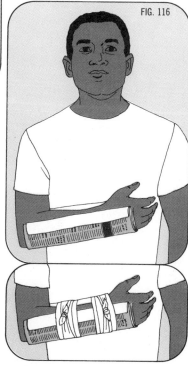

FIG. 116

keeping his thumb pointing upward (Fig. 117). Observe the precautions noted above. If an air splint is used (Fig. 118), follow the instructions that accompany it. Take particular care to avoid overinflation, which may result in a critical reduction in blood circulation.

A common fracture of the lower end of the radius, called a Colles fracture, occurs just above the wrist and often produces backward angulation of the hand. This injury is generally the result of a fall with the wrist bent backward beyond the normal range of motion.

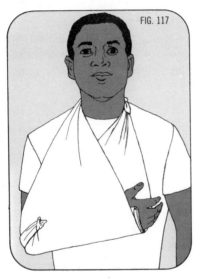

FIG. 117

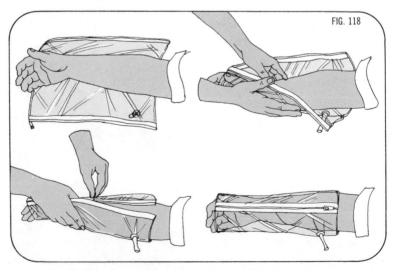

FIG. 118

This fracture is extremely painful and, like all major fractures, may precipitate shock. Have the victim lie down. He will be more comfortable if he supports his injured arm with his other hand until splints are applied. Place his forearm on a pillow (Fig. 119) and apply well-padded splints. Check to see that ties are not too tight. Then bend his elbow (Fig. 120) and have him rest his forearm on his chest or apply a sling, whichever is more comfortable. Check his fingers repeatedly; if swelling develops, loosen the ties of the splint.

Fracture of one of the eight small bones that make up the wrist is often difficult to detect and may be misdiagnosed as a sprain. First aid consists of splinting and elevation. Place a padded board under the victim's forearm, wrist, and hand, and secure it in a position so that his wrist cannot be moved in any direction.

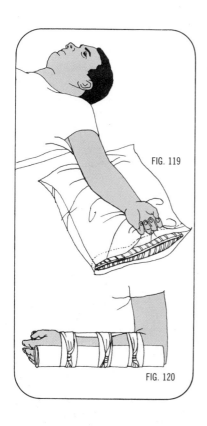

FIG. 119

FIG. 120

Hand and Fingers (Fig. 121)

Fractures of the bones of the hand are common, particularly at the knuckles. They are seen most often in the little finger as a result

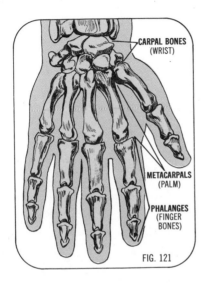

CARPAL BONES
(WRIST)

METACARPALS
(PALM)

PHALANGES
(FINGER
BONES)

FIG. 121

of a blow inflicted in fighting; the small bones of the fingers are also vulnerable to injury, both singly and in combination with other fractures. First aid for a fracture of a single finger consists of splinting with a small padded board or metal strip with the finger in a comfortable position. For a severe crushing injury, do not cleanse the wound. Place a ball of gauze or a pad of cloth in the victim's palm and cover his entire hand with a large pad or bulky cover of clean linen, which will help to splint the hand and make him more comfortable. To relieve pain and to minimize harmful effects to the delicate structures of the hand and fingers produced by swelling, the first-aider must keep the injured hand raised at all times, on pillows if necessary, and the hand should *never* be allowed to hang down.

Hip and Thigh (Fig. 122)

Fractures of the hip joint involving the upper portion of the femur, the thigh bone, commonly result from falls and automobile accidents. Owing to the heavy muscular coverage, there is seldom an open fracture in this location, but bleeding into the tissues, often severe, may produce shock.

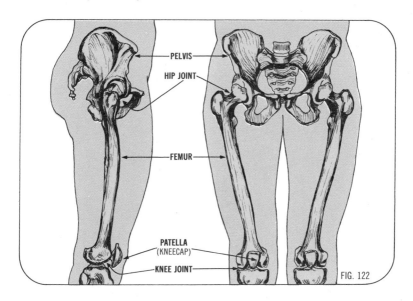

PELVIS

HIP JOINT

FEMUR

PATELLA
(KNEECAP)

KNEE JOINT

FIG. 122

An impacted fracture in the hip may be the result of very slight injury in an older person. In this case, the two ends of the bone are pushed together rather than apart. There may be only moderate pain and mild disability at first, so that the victim may even be able to bear weight. But bearing weight must be avoided if there is any chance that a fracture has occurred. It is important, therefore, to advise that a physician be consulted about an X-ray examination if there is pain in the victim's hip region and a limp on the affected side.

Fractures of the shaft of the femur usually result from falls or traffic injuries. The victim is in severe pain and shock, as a rule, and markedly disabled. His foot is characteristically turned outward and the limb shortened, owing to overlapping of the bone ends due to muscular spasm. If the victim is to be transported only a short distance on a stretcher, place a blanket between his legs and bind them together. If you use improvised board splints, they should be well padded and should reach from the victim's armpit to below his heel on the outer side of the leg and from the groin (also protected by pad) on the inner side of the leg (Fig. 123). To apply the board splint, assemble needed supplies (Fig. 124). Push cravat bandages— or strips of cloth—under the victim at the ankle, the knee, and the lower back (see page 174, Fig. 107E). Slide bandages into place (Fig. 125). Place padded splints in position (Fig. 126). Place additional padding at the knee and ankle. Complete by making snug ties on the outer splint (Figs. 127 and 128). Place ties at his chest, flank, groin, knee, and ankle. If an open wound is present, do not attempt to cleanse it; cover it with a sterile or clean bulky pad after cutting away contaminated clothing, apply pressure through it to control hemorrhage, secure the dressing in place, and splint.

If at all possible, apply a traction splint at the scene of the accident for fractures of the shaft of the femur. This splint will provide the best fixation of the fracture and make the victim comfortable, but only persons with specific training in the application of traction splints should attempt to apply it (see page 194).

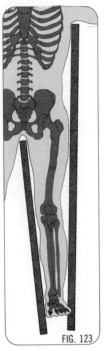

FIG. 123

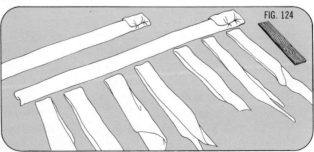

FIG. 124

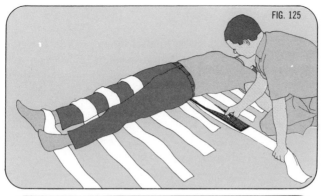

FIG. 125

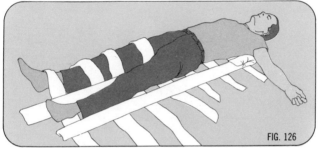

FIG. 126

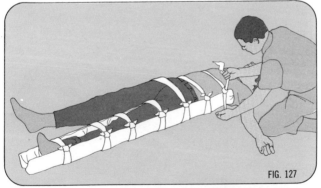

FIG. 127

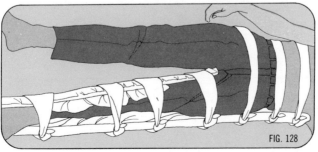

FIG. 128

Kneecap (Fig. 130)

The kneecap, or patella, is in front of the knee joint. It is fractured usually by a direct blow or in injuries sustained when control of the knee is lost, with the front thigh muscles pulling violently on the kneecap. As <u>first aid</u>, apply a pillow or blanket splint or padded splints from below the victim's heel to his buttocks along the back of the leg, with the leg extended (Fig. 129).

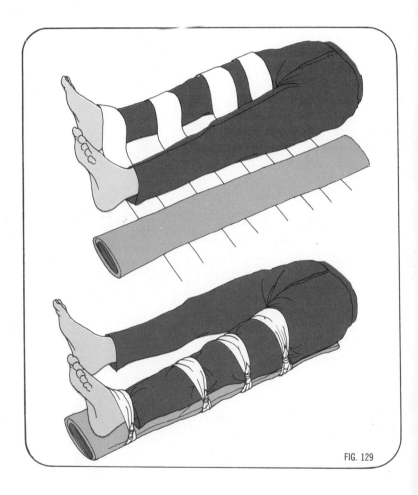

FIG. 129

Lower Leg (Fig. 130)

The bones of the lower leg are the tibia, or shinbone, which supports the weight of the body and may be felt directly beneath the skin along the front of the leg, and the slender fibula on the outer side. The fibula forms the outside wall of the ankle. Fractures of these bones occur often. A common type of fracture at the upper end of the tibia just below the knee joint is the so-called bumper fracture, sustained by a pedestrian who is hit on the outer surface of his leg by an automobile bumper. Fractures of the shaft are often associated with open wounds, because the bone is covered only by skin and a thin layer of tissue beneath it.

An uncomplicated break in the fibula alone is often not recognized if the victim has minimal pain. Because this bone does not bear weight and is splinted naturally by the tibia, the victim can walk and might not seek medical care until swelling and persistent pain cause him concern.

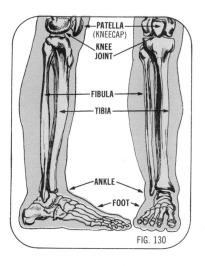

FIG. 130

First aid for fractures of the tibia and fibula consists of applying well-padded splints on both sides of the leg and foot (Fig. 131); applying a padded, three-sided box splint of cardboard on the entire leg and foot; or, in an emergency, inserting blankets or towels between the victim's legs and tying the legs together. Remember to keep the victim's foot pointing upward, and check constantly to make sure that bandages do not interfere with circulation to his lower leg and foot.

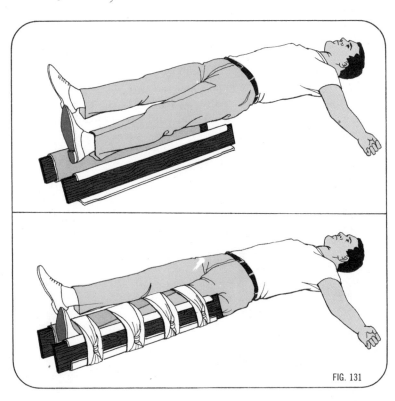

FIG. 131

Ankle and Foot (Fig. 132)

The ankle is made up of the lower ends of the tibia and fibula and first bone of the foot (the talus). Six bones make up the back half of the foot; the front half comprises the five metatarsal bones and the toes. Fractures of the foot ordinarily result from direct injury: twisting, being run over, or being hit by a heavy object. The heel bone, or

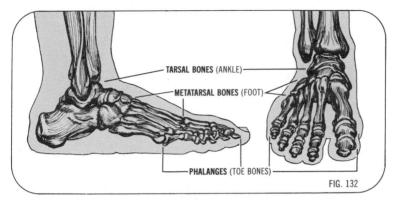

TARSAL BONES (ANKLE)

METATARSAL BONES (FOOT)

PHALANGES (TOE BONES)

FIG. 132

calcaneus, may be fractured if a person jumps or falls from a height while in a standing position. The metatarsals and the small bones of the toes may be broken by stubbing or twisting the toes or as the result of falling objects or a crushing injury. "March fractures" of the metatarsals, seen in young adults after prolonged walking, are fine cracks in the bone where there has been no history of obvious injury.

In first aid for fractures of the feet, remove the victim's shoes and hose and keep him lying down with his leg elevated. For an open wound, apply large, bulky dressings, sterile if possible. Splint with a pillow, firmly applied, without attempting to correct the deformity (Fig. 133).

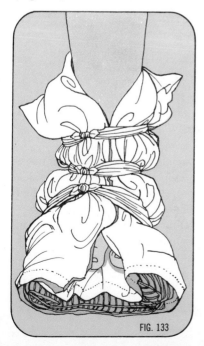

FIG. 133

DISLOCATIONS

A dislocation is a displacement of a bone end from the joint—particularly in the shoulder (Fig. 134A), elbow, fingers, or thumb (Fig. 134B)—usually as a result of a fall or a direct blow. There is usually swelling, obvious deformity, and pain. The first aid worker

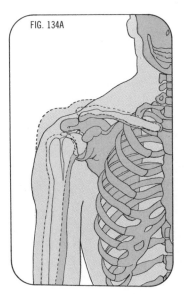

FIG. 134A

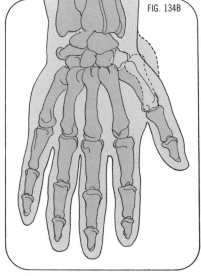

FIG. 134B

should *not* attempt to reduce a dislocation or to correct any deformity near a joint, because often extensive tearing of the joint capsule has occurred, and careless handling may cause additional tearing of supportive structures and, at the same time, injure blood vessels and nerves in the area.

First aid should be essentially the same as for closed fractures: splinting and immobilizing the affected joint in the position in which it is found; applying a sling, if appropriate; elevating the affected part, if a limb is involved; and securing medical attention promptly.

Dislocation of one of the intervertebral disks of fibrous cartilage in the lumbar region or in the neck results from protrusion of the disk backward into the spinal canal through a weakened or ruptured ligament. Symptoms are due to pressure on the spinal cord, either on the side or on the midline. Characteristically, the victim gives a history of episodes of pain, accentuated by coughing, sneezing, or straining; of muscle weakness and spasm; and of disturbances in sensation, such as numbness and tingling. Pain in the back often extends along the course of the sciatic nerve down the back of the victim's leg. A cervical disk produces shoulder and arm pain that radiates down the arm. At times, acute back or neck pain may develop suddenly after the victim lifts a heavy weight or after he suffers some other injury, in which case fracture of the spine may be suspected. First aid is the same as for other spinal injuries: Summon an ambulance with proper transportation equipment; do not move the victim without adequate help and a backboard support to maintain proper alignment of his body; and avoid twisting and forward and backward bending of the victim's spine.

In addition to dislocation of bones of the knee joint, dislocation or tearing of the fibrocartilage in the knee (occasionally in other joints as well) results from a fall, from an accident while the victim is kneeling, or from a twisting injury while the victim is engaged in a rigorous sport. The knee may lock as the cartilage is displaced from its position at the margin of the joint to a location between the ends of the femur and the tibia. First aid is the same as for a fracture. Do *not* attempt to straighten the leg.

SPRAINS

Sprains, injuries to the soft tissues surrounding joints, usually result from motion forced beyond the normal range at a joint. The ligaments, tendons, and blood vessels are stretched and occasionally torn or partially torn.

Sprains are particularly common about the ankle, usually from turning the foot inward beyond the normal range of motion, and in the knee, from a wrenching movement or a direct blow. Wrist sprains are less common, and fractures of the fingers may be mistaken for sprains.

Sprains of the neck result from falls, from injuries occurring in sports such as football, and from automobile accidents in which a stationary or slowly moving car is suddenly struck from behind. The victim's body is jerked forward, and his unsupported head is violently thrust backward and then forward (whiplash). Part of the pain and disability in this and other types of sprains is due to muscle strain or overstretching, as well as to injury to the ligaments.

It is usually impossible to distinguish a severe sprain from a fracture without X-ray examination. (For information on neck injuries, see page 164).

First aid for sprains is as follows:

- If the victim's ankle or knee is affected, do not allow him to walk.
- Apply a pillow splint or a blanket splint by forming a horseshoe around the injured foot (Figs. 135 and 136). Tie snugly with strips

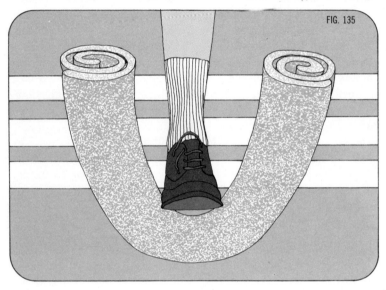

FIG. 135

of cloth or cravat bandages located below the ankle (around heel), at the ankle, and above the ankle (Fig. 137). Elevate the victim's

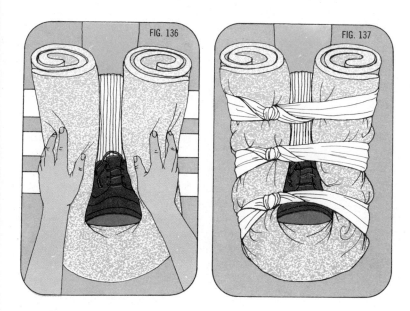

leg, because swelling may produce greater disability than the original injury itself.

- In mild sprains, keep the injured part raised for at least 24 hours. Do *not* soak in *hot* water. Apply cold, wet packs, or place a small bag of crushed ice on the affected area, over a thin towel to protect the victim's skin. Packs may be applied over a period of several days. Do not pack the joint in ice, and do not immerse the injured limb in water that contains ice.
- If swelling and pain persist, seek medical attention.

STRAINS

Strains are injuries to muscles from overexertion. The fibers are stretched and sometimes partially torn.

A strain is often confused with a sprain and at times with other injuries, such as a "charley horse" of the leg, an injury that is common in sports and is generally due to a small hemorrhage in the deep tissues. The most extensive strain involves the back muscles.

This disability is usually the result of lifting something improperly or of lifting an object that is too heavy. It often incapacitates the victim for a long period. All severe back strains should be seen by a physician for diagnosis and treatment and for clearance before the person returns to physical labor.

First aid for a strained back consists of bed rest, heat, and use of a board under the mattress for firm support. First aid for other strains consists of application of heat, warm, wet applications, and rest.

APPLICATION OF TRACTION SPLINTS FOR FRACTURE OF THE FEMUR

The best emergency treatment for a fracture of the femur is the application of a traction splint. Such a splint not only immobilizes the injured part but also helps to minimize overlapping of the bone fragments, which occurs from spasm of muscles adjacent to the fracture location. The amount of overlap, or overriding, varies considerably but it may be as much as 2 inches, or even more. Most overriding occurs at once as a result of the forces that produce the fracture, but overriding can increase over a period of several hours.

Muscle spasm also causes broken ends of bone to injure muscles, blood vessels, and nerves in the area. Motion by the injured person or movement associated with transportation may increase overriding and injuries to other structures. A traction splint keeps the body part immobile, thus minimizing injury to the soft tissues from the sharp bone ends. Although the splint does not relieve all spasm and pain, it will lessen the tendency for overriding to increase.

The half-ring traction splint (which is called a Keller-Blake splint) is exceptionally useful, particularly for a fracture of the thigh. First aid students who expect to work as ambulance attendants, as firefighters, in rescue squads, or in industrial first aid rooms should familiarize themselves with the application of the splint and practice repeatedly in two-man teams.

Half-Ring Splint

1. Prepare the splint for use. First, make a cravat bandage. Bring the two ends together and lay the loop over the end of the splint (Fig. 138). Bring the two tails through the loop (Fig. 139) and pull downward to tighten (Fig. 140). Make sure the ends of the bandage are of equal length. This procedure completes the splint lock hitch.
2. Apply a sprained ankle bandage. Place the middle of a narrow cravat under the shoe, just in front of the heel. Carry the ends

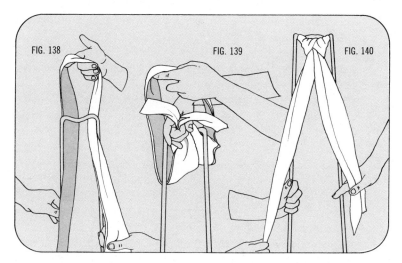

FIG. 138   FIG. 139   FIG. 140

up and back, crossing them at the back of the heel (Fig. 141A). Continue around the ankle, crossing the ends over the instep (Fig. 141B), then downward toward the arch to make a hitch under the cravat on each side, in front of the heel (Fig. 141C). Pull the ends in opposite directions to achieve the desired tension. Cross the ends over the instep and tie them (Fig. 141D).

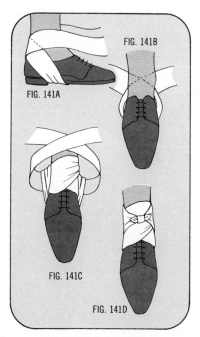

FIG. 141A
FIG. 141B
FIG. 141C
FIG. 141D

The bandage should be snug but not tight and as free of wrinkles as possible.

3. Direct a helper to grasp the foot of the limb to be splinted with one of his hands over the instep and the other at the lower part of the heel and to exert a strong, steady pull as the foot is elevated sufficiently for the splint and cravat bandages to be properly applied by other helpers (Fig. 142). The helper should maintain traction on the foot until the limb is splinted and all ties are completed. (If a fragment of bone is protruding through the skin, care should be taken not to apply so much traction that the end of the broken bone will be pulled back into the depths of the wound.)

4. Flatten the half-ring on the splint and slip it in place underneath the injured limb, with the long bar of the splint on the outer side of the limb and the half-ring resting against the victim's buttocks. Using the straps, lift the half-ring into place against the victim's buttocks and fasten it loosely over his thigh. Allow enough room between the strap and the thigh to pass your fingers through easily (Fig. 143).

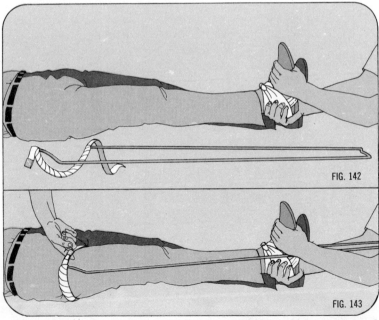

FIG. 142

FIG. 143

5. Pass the ends of the lock hitch downward through the stirrups of the ankle bandage and around the bars of the splint (Fig. 144). Before tying both ends around the bars of the splint, make sure that you have equaled the tension maintained by the helper who is holding the foot in position.

6. Insert a short, strong stick between the ends, running from the end of the splint to the foot (Fig. 145) and twist it until the desired amount of traction is attained, so that there will be no release of traction when the hands are removed (Fig. 146). Then tie the stick to the sides of the splint so that it will not unwind.

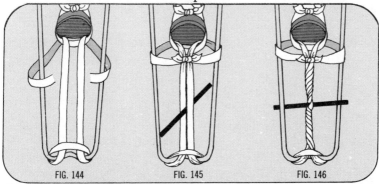

FIG. 144   FIG. 145   FIG. 146

7. Use cravat bandages to form cradle hitches, which will act as a hammock to support the injured limb from the ankle to the groin. To apply a cradle hitch, hang the cravat over the bar. Next pass the end nearest the leg under the leg, up between the leg and the inside bar. Pass the second half of the cravat under and around the leg and both side bars. Then pull the ends in opposite directions to bring the limb into a comfortable position. Place a cradle hitch under the suspected site of fracture to support it and prevent angulation of the bone ends.
(NOTE. A sufficient number of cradle hitches must be applied to assure support of the entire limb (Figs. 147 and 148).

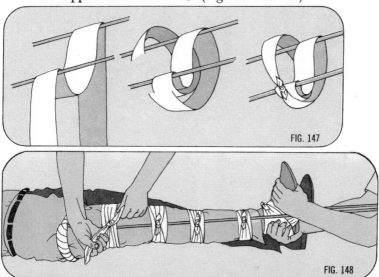

FIG. 147

FIG. 148

8. Place a block under the end of the splint to prevent the heel from coming into contact with the ground or cot. If a foot support for the splint is available, secure the toe of the shoe to the wire with a cravat bandage.
9. Direct helper to release traction.
10. During transportation, make sure the heel is supported so that there is no pressure on it.
11. Check circular ties often to make sure that they are not too tight.

Lock Hitch for Notched-Board Splint

To attach traction bands to a *notched board*, fold a cravat bandage in the middle and lay about 8 inches of this fold through the notch (Fig. 149A). Open the loop at the fold and double the open loop back over the ends of the notch (Fig. 149B). Pull the ends of the cravat until the loop is snug (Fig. 149C).

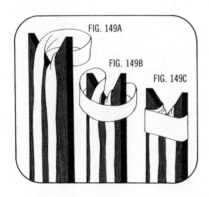

FIG. 149A

FIG. 149B

FIG. 149C

Lock Hitch for Plain Board

To attach traction bands to an unnotched board, start with a wide cravat bandage. Tie a loose overhand (half) knot, separating the loops to form an opening (Fig. 150A). Place this opening over the end of the board, bringing it down until the end of the board catches in the middle of the cravat (Fig. 150B). Pull the ends of the cravat in opposite directions (Fig. 150C) until taut (Fig. 150D). This same procedure is used to tie the lock hitch on a stick (Fig. 151). A loose overhand knot over the end of a stick or board may also be used (Fig. 152).

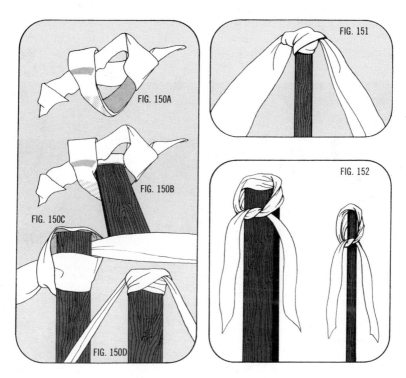

Improvised Fixed-Traction Splint

An improvised splint can be made with a board about 5 feet long, 4 inches wide, and 1/2 inch thick. A V-shaped notch should be cut in each end of the board.

1. Put on a sprained ankle bandage (see page 195, Figs. 141A through 141D).
2. Apply manual traction on the foot (see page 196, Fig. 142).
3. Slip a second cravat under the leg and slide it up the leg until the center of the bandage is in the crotch. Then tie the ends so that a

loop is formed above the hip into which the notch of the upper end of the board is placed. Secure the cravat in the notch with the tails of the bandage (Fig. 153).

4. Insert the tails of the lock hitch downward through the stirrups of the sprained ankle bandage, pass them over and under the board (Fig. 154A), and tie them (Fig. 154B).

5. Insert a stout, strong stick between the traction bands below the foot and twist it until you have taken up any slack left while tying the traction bands around the splint (Figs. 154C and 155).

6. Place padding between the leg and the board wherever pressure occurs.

7. Wrap several *wide* cravats around the limb and board from the ankle to the upper thigh (Fig. 156).

8. Support the end of the splint so that the heel does not come into contact with the ground.

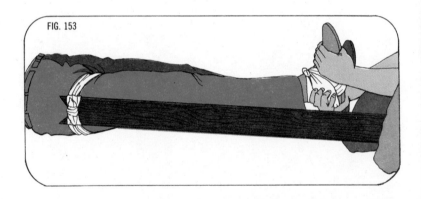

FIG. 153

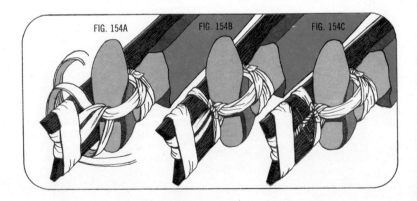

FIG. 154A   FIG. 154B   FIG. 154C

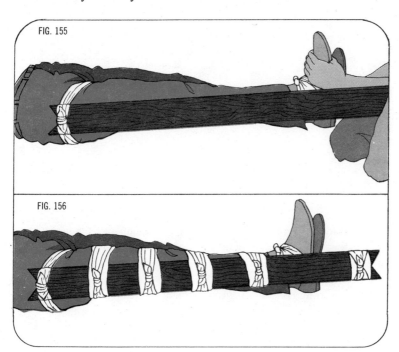

FIG. 155

FIG. 156

14

DRESSINGS AND BANDAGES

Techniques of applying dressings and bandages vary according to the extent and location of injuries, the material at hand, and the ability of the first-aider to adapt to an emergency situation. Supplies can be obtained commercially for home use, or substitutes can be prepared from household linen. It may be necessary to improvise dressings and bandages from any woven fabric available, or even from facial tissues, other paper goods, or unused plastic bags. Fluff cotton, which may be used to pad a splint, should never be placed directly upon an open wound, because the fibers are difficult to remove.

DEFINITIONS

Dressings

A dressing, also called a compress, is an immediate protective cover placed over a wound to assist in the control of hemorrhage, to absorb blood and wound secretions, to prevent additional contamination, and to ease pain. Sterile dressings are those free from germs before use.

A sterile dressing is preferable, but if it is not obtainable, a freshly ironed or laundered cloth—such as a handkerchief, towel, sheet, pillowcase, or napkin—may be used.

To sterilize dressings at home, wrap them in aluminum foil and place them in a moderate oven (350° F) for 3 hours, or boil them for 15 minutes and dry them without contamination. For immediate use, a clean cloth pressed with a hot iron or the inner surface of a folded cloth will usually suffice. Do not touch, breathe on, or cough on the surface of a dressing that is to be placed next to a wound.

Use a dressing large enough to extend an inch or more beyond the edge of the wound. First hold it over the wound and then lower it into place; do not slide it onto the wound from the side. If a dressing slips off onto surrounding skin before it has been anchored in place, discard it. Secure a dressing with bandages or tape, but *do not* wrap tape completely around the affected part, because blood vessels may be constricted as swelling occurs.

Bandages

A bandage is a strip of woven material used to hold a wound dressing or splint in place. It helps to immobilize, support, and protect an injured part of the body. Occasionally, large pieces of cloth are used as bandages, slings, and binders.

A bandage must be clean but need not be sterile. The most useful of those available commercially (Fig. 157) include—

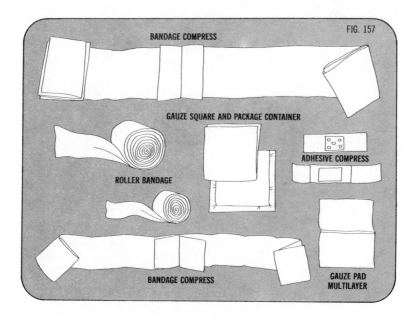

FIG. 157

BANDAGE COMPRESS

GAUZE SQUARE AND PACKAGE CONTAINER

ADHESIVE COMPRESS

ROLLER BANDAGE

BANDAGE COMPRESS

GAUZE PAD MULTILAYER

- Gauze bandages, usually in rolls 10 yards long and 1, 2, or 3 inches wide.
- Elastic bandages of woven material in various widths and lengths.
- Triangular bandages, usually of muslin, approximately 55 inches across at the base and from 36 to 40 inches along the sides. These bandages are included in first aid kits and are useful as covering

for large areas, as slings, and, when folded lengthwise, as cravat bandages (see page 207, Figs. 158A through 158D). They also can be folded into thick pads for pressure over a wound to control hemorrhage.

• Binders of muslin, to be applied to the chest (see page 212, Fig. 173) or abdomen. (A large towel or part of a sheet can substitute for a binder. Binders are rarely used except as emergency bandages or dressings to cover large areas of the trunk, such as the chest or abdomen. A binder may be pinned in place or held with several ties or cravat bandages. Great care must be taken not to apply a binder so tightly that it interferes with breathing.)

Other emergency bandages can be devised from handkerchiefs, household linen, belts, ties, socks, or stockings. Bandages can be held in place with adhesive, with plastic or masking tape, with safety pins, or with clips. Gauze and muslin bandages can be split and tied.

Combination Dressings and Bandages

Adhesive strips with gauze dressings attached are available commercially in a wide variety of sizes and shapes. Another useful dressing-bandage combination is the *bandage compress*, which is usually included in the supplies of a first aid kit. It consists of a pad made of several thicknesses of sterile gauze sewed to the middle of a strip of gauze or muslin. Bandage compresses are the most useful and efficient combination of bandage and dressing to apply to a large wound as an emergency cover. The dressing portion provides bulk over which pressure may be applied for control of severe hemorrhage. If desired, it can be converted into a four-tail bandage compress by splitting each end of the gauze or muslin toward the center, leaving a pocket that can be positioned around an irregular surface, such as the chin, the heel, or a joint region.

Special Pads

Large, thick, layered pads with a waterproofed outer surface are available in several sizes for rapid application to a limb or a large area of the trunk. Because they are often used in the treatment of persons with circular burns, they are sometimes called "burn pads" or "general-purpose dressings." They are also used without bandages for patients to lie on in bed when a thick, absorbent dressing that can be changed quickly with minimal discomfort is desired.

USE OF BANDAGES AND DRESSINGS

A bandage should be snug (it is useless if too loose) but not so tight as to interfere with circulation, either at the time of application or later if swelling occurs. Bandages that are too tight may cause permanent damage to blood vessels, nerves, and other tissue—even paralysis and gangrene. For this reason, leave a person's fingertips exposed when you apply a splint or bandage to his arm, and leave his toes exposed when you apply a splint or bandage to his leg. Watch for swelling, changes of color, and coldness of the tips of fingers or toes, which would indicate interference with circulation. Loosen bandages immediately if the patient complains of numbness or a tingling sensation.

Never apply a tight circular bandage about a person's neck; it may cause strangulation. To secure a dressing in the jaw region, apply one turn of a bandage and tie the ends with a bow knot on top of the person's head, so that the bandage can be removed quickly if he vomits.

Elastic Bandages

In using elastic bandages, be very careful not to stretch the material too tightly. Although they are the easiest of all bandages to apply and are especially useful, because they conform more readily to an injured part than gauze or muslin, elastic bandages are also the most hazardous because of the first-aider's tendency to stretch them so much that they impair circulation or nerve function. They are rather expensive but can be laundered and used repeatedly for a number of purposes.

To apply an elastic bandage, begin at the lower portion of the area to be covered and, after one or two circular turns, proceed upward; overlap succeeding turns by approximately 1/2 to 3/4 of an inch. Use metal clips, tape, or small safety pins to secure the ends.

At the ankle, knee, elbow, wrist, and shoulder, the bandage should be applied in a figure-of-eight (see page 215, Figs. 181A through 181F, and page 218, Figs. 188A and 188B) for better fit and support. This configuration also can be used for wounds of the thigh and groin areas, with circular turns about the waist. To apply the bandage on the head or over an eye patch, make one or two circular turns, first horizontally across the forehead and then diagonally across the scalp, to hold the dressing in place.

Gauze Bandages

Skill is necessary in applying a gauze bandage to prevent its slipping and stretching, because gauze is very loosely woven. Never apply a wet gauze bandage. As it dries, it will shrink and become too tight. Gauze can be used to bandage almost any part of the body. Choose the appropriate width. The most common uses are for—

- Circular bandages.
- Spiral bandages.
- Figure-of-eight bandages (for joint areas).
- Fingertip bandages (formerly called recurrent), which are applied with several circular turns, then a number of loops perpendicular to these turns to cover the tip of the finger, and, finally, additional circular turns to hold the loops firmly in place (see pages 220 and 221, Figs. 191A through 191D and Figs. 192A through 192C).

Triangular Bandages

A triangular bandage is useful as an emergency cover for a person's entire scalp, hand, or foot, or for any large area. Such a bandage is used also as a sling for a fracture or other injury of an arm or hand. Folded into a cravat bandage (*cravat* means necktie), a triangle can be used as a circular, spiral, or figure-of-eight bandage as a tie for a splint, as a constricting band, as a tourniquet; and, if the cravat bandage is folded several times again to form a thick pad, as an emergency dressing for control of bleeding or over another dressing to provide protection and pressure.

Triangular Bandage Folded as Cravat

To make a cravat, bring the point of a triangular bandage to the middle of the base (Figs. 158A and 158B). Then fold lengthwise along the middle until you obtain the desired width (Figs. 158C and 158D).

Adhesive-Strip Dressings

Adhesive-strip dressings or homemade substitutes are used for small wounds, after the wounds have been thoroughly cleansed. Blot the skin surface dry before applying the tape. Hold the edges of a cut together as the dressing is secured in place.

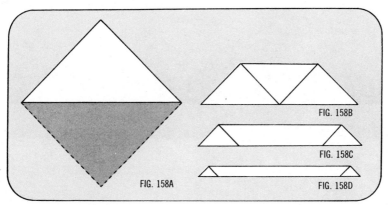

FIG. 158B

FIG. 158C

FIG. 158A

FIG. 158D

Bandage-Anchoring

Place the end of the bandage on a bias at the starting point (Fig. 159). Encircle the part, allowing the corner of the bandage end to protrude (Fig. 160). Turn down the protruding tip of the bandage and encircle the part again (Figs. 161 and 162).

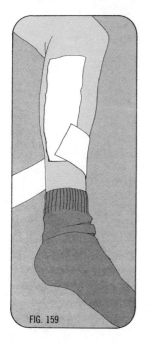

FIG. 159

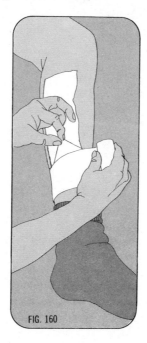

FIG. 160

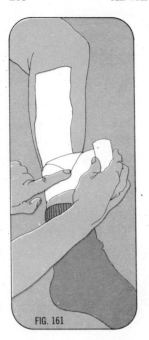

FIG. 161

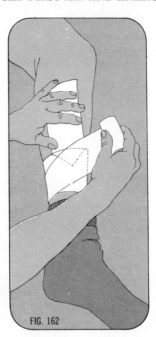

FIG. 162

Bandage-Securing

Several ways to secure a bandage in place were mentioned on page 204. Another method for tying gauze or muslin in place is illustrated below.

Take the bandage end in a direction away from the body part being covered; loop it around your thumb or finger and continue back to the opposite side of the body part (Fig. 163); encircle the part with the looped end and the free end and tie them together (Fig. 164).

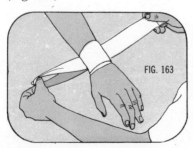

FIG. 163

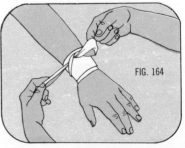

FIG. 164

BANDAGES FOR SPECIFIC PURPOSES

Open Triangular Bandage for Scalp and Forehead

Fold a hem about 2 inches wide along the base. Place compress. Put the dressing in place with the hem on the outside. Place the bandage on the head so that the middle of the base lies on the forehead close to the eyebrows, with the point hanging down in back (Fig. 165A). Carry the two ends around the head above the ears and cross (do not tie) them, just below the bump at the back of the head (Fig. 165B). Draw the ends snug, carry them around the

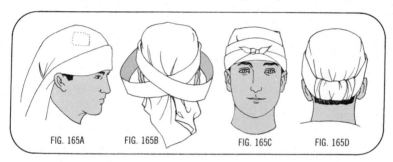

FIG. 165A   FIG. 165B   FIG. 165C   FIG. 165D

head, and tie them in the center of the forehead (Fig. 165C). Steady the head with one hand, and with the other, draw the point down firmly behind to hold the compress securely against the head. Pick up the point and tuck it in where the bandage ends cross (Fig. 165D) or pin it with a safety pin at the back of the head.

Cravat Bandage for Forehead, Ears, or Eyes

Place the center of the cravat over the compress that covers the wound (Fig. 166A). Carry the ends around to the opposite side of the head and cross them (Fig. 166B). Bring them back to the starting point and tie them (Fig. 166C).

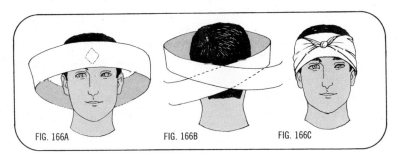

FIG. 166A   FIG. 166B   FIG. 166C

Cravat Bandage for Cheek, Ear, or Head

Use a wide cravat. Start with the middle of the cravat over the compress that covers the cheek or ear (Fig. 167A). Carry one end over the top of the head and the other under the chin. Cross the ends at the opposite side, bringing the short end back around the forehead and the long end around the back of the head (Fig. 167B). Tie them over the compress (Fig. 167C). Never use this method for a fracture of the jaw or when there is bleeding in the mouth or danger of vomiting, unless an attendant will be constantly present to loosen the bandage in an emergency.

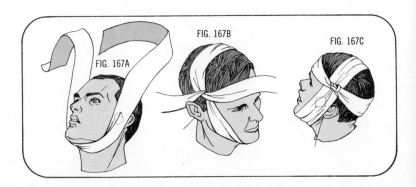

FIG. 167A   FIG. 167B   FIG. 167C

Four-Tail Bandage for Face or Jaw

The appearance of this bandage gives it its name. Because a pocket can be formed by crossing the tails in pairs when tying the bandage, the bandage fits particularly well over protuberances, such as the nose and chin. A piece of cloth about 3 feet long and from 3 to 8 inches wide is split from each end down the middle, leaving as large a center area as is needed. Gauze may be used, but heavier cloth is more satisfactory. First apply a dressing over the wound, then center the bandage over it. The two upper tails are tied together at the back (Fig. 168A), and the two lower tails are tied at the top of the head (Fig. 168B), so that the bandage fits smoothly (Fig. 168C). This bandage may be used for wounds of the nose, chin, and lower jaw (Figs. 169A through 169C)—but only on a conscious victim.

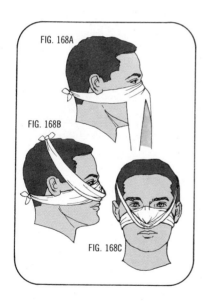

FIG. 168A

FIG. 168B

FIG. 168C

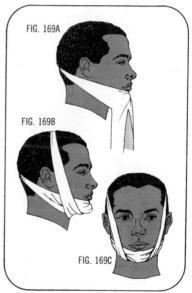

FIG. 169A

FIG. 169B

FIG. 169C

Triangular Bandage for Chest or Back

Place the point of the bandage over the shoulder on the injured side. With the dressing in place, bring the bandage down over the chest (or back) so that the middle of the base is directly below the point. Roll or fold the base as far up as you desire. Carry the ends around the body (Fig. 170). Tie them directly below the shoulder (Fig. 171). One long and one short end will be left. Lift the long end up to the shoulder and tie it to the point of the triangle (Fig. 172).

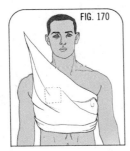
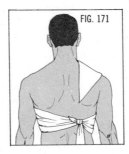
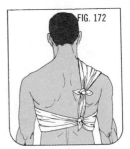

Muslin Binder for Chest or Abdomen

When bulky dressings are needed for wounds of the abdomen or chest, the simplest form of bandage is usually a binder, made from a rectangular piece of muslin or other cloth from 12 to 18 inches wide and from 3 to 5 feet long. The binder is placed around the back and pinned in front (Fig. 173). A large bath towel makes a good binder.

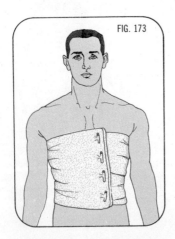

Triangular Bandage for Shoulder or Hip

Two triangular bandages, or one triangular bandage and a necktie or strip of cloth, are required. If two triangular bandages are used, fold one into a narrow cravat. Pin or roll the point of the second (unfolded) triangular bandage around this cravat several turns to secure it. Pleat the unfolded triangular bandage, laying it with the middle of the folded cravat over the injured shoulder. Bring the end of the cravat or strip of cloth around the body below the opposite armpit and tie it slightly forward from the armpit (Fig. 174). Unfold the pleated triangle, bringing it down over the dressing so that the base of the bandage lies on the arm (Fig. 175). Fold the bandage up the arm as far as desired. Wrap the ends around the arm and tie them snugly (Fig. 176). Check the pulse at the wrist on the injured side to make sure that circulation has not been reduced. The same procedure is used for bandaging the hip (Fig. 177).

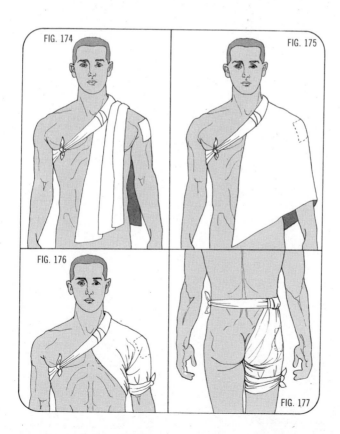

FIG. 174 FIG. 175 FIG. 176 FIG. 177

Figure-of-Eight Bandage for Neck and Armpit

Make two or more anchoring wraps around the arm. Bring the bandage from under the armpit, upward and diagonally across the shoulder (Fig. 178), behind the neck, around to the front of the neck, diagonally downward, behind the same shoulder, and then under the armpit (Fig. 179). Repeat figure-of-eight turns several times, so that by overlapping you can cover the dressing and hold it in place. Complete by tying off (Fig. 180).

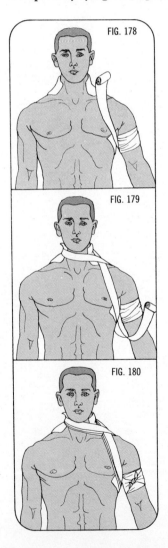

FIG. 178

FIG. 179

FIG. 180

Figure-of-Eight Bandage for Elbow or Knee

This application is basically the same as that used for the neck and armpit (Figs. 178 through 180)—circular turns connected by diagonal crossings at the joint. Make several anchoring turns, overlapping the top edge of the dressing (Fig. 181A). Proceed diagonally across the dressing (Fig. 181B). Circle below the joint (Fig. 181C) and diagonally back across the dressing (Fig. 181D) to complete the figure-of-eight (Fig. 181E). Repeat the figure-of-eight process until the area is sufficiently covered (Fig. 181F). Complete by tying off. This turn may be used on the elbow and other angular surfaces of the body.

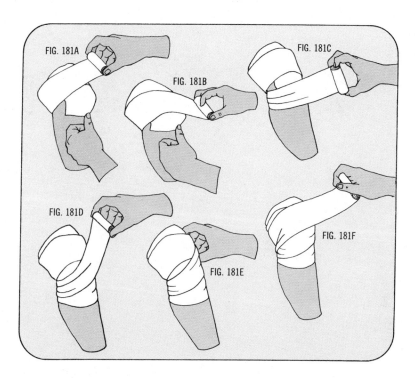

Cravat Bandage for Elbow or Knee

Bend the elbow or knee at a right angle, unless this movement produces pain. Use a rather wide bandage (Fig. 182A). Start with the middle of the bandage over the dressing at the elbow or knee (Fig. 182B). Carry the ends around in opposite directions (one end around the upper arm or leg and the other around the lower part), crossing them in the hollow (Fig. 182C). Continue the bandage around, covering the dressing. Carry it back to the hollow and tie on the outside of the limb (Figs. 182D and 182E).

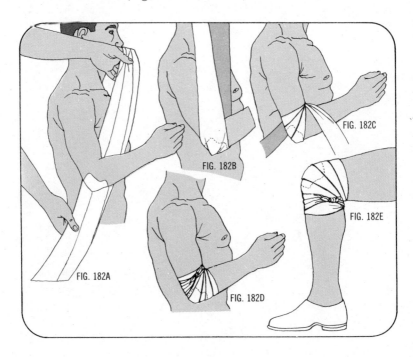

FIG. 182C

FIG. 182B

FIG. 182E

FIG. 182A

FIG. 182D

Open and Closed Spiral Bandage of a Limb

Begin by anchoring as previously described (see page 207). Continue to encircle the area to be covered, using spiral turns spaced so that they do not overlap (Figs. 183 and 184). Complete the bandage by tying off (Fig. 185). This bandage may be useful as a temporary bandage, for splinting, and to hold a large burn dressing in place. It may be closed (closed spiral) simply by continuing to encircle with

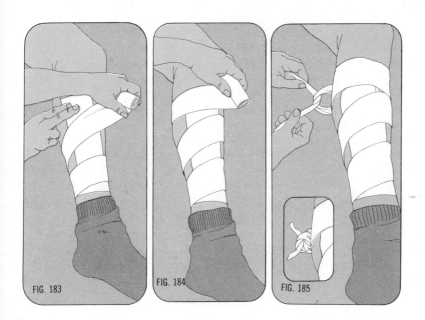

FIG. 183   FIG. 184   FIG. 185

spiral turns until all the gaps are closed. This method of application for the closed spiral bandage will achieve the same result as the spiral reverse described below.

Spiral Reverse Bandage of a Limb

Because the limbs are tapered, a spiral bandage sometimes must include an occasional reverse-lap to fill gaps in the bandage. Anchor the bandage. Take two or three turns around the small part of the limb. Then start wrapping with a spiral turn as long as each turn will lie flat and overlap the preceding turn by at least one-third the width of the bandage. When a gap develops, it requires a "reverse."

Hold the lower edge of the last turn that fits properly, then loosely make a neat half-twist or lap to slightly change the direction of the spiral (Fig. 186). Continue the spiral wrap up the limb, repeating the "reverse" each time it is needed (Fig. 187).

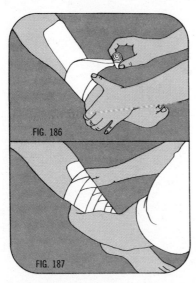

Figure-of-Eight Bandage for Hand and Wrist

Anchor the bandage with one or more turns around the palm of the hand. Carry it diagonally across the back of the hand and then around the wrist (Figs. 188A and 188B). Again carry it diagonally across the back of the hand and back to the palm. This figure-of-eight maneuver is repeated as many times as is necessary to fix the dressing properly. Complete by tying off.

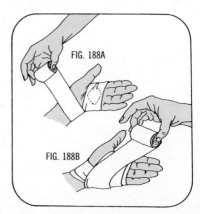

Bandage Compress

Place the compress (pad) directly over the wound (Fig. 189A). Encircle by taking the ends of the bandage around in opposite directions (Fig. 189B), and continue to encircle until the wrist is sufficiently covered. Tie off (Fig. 189C). Although shown on the wrist, the bandage compress is applicable to all circular parts of the body (arms, legs, chest, etc.). For a further description of the bandage compress, see page 204.

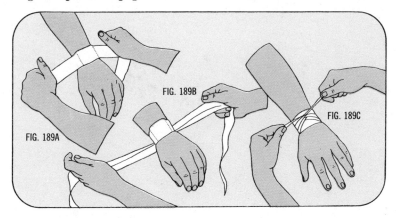

FIG. 189A   FIG. 189B   FIG. 189C

Pressure Bandage for Palm

Place a sterile pad in the palm of the hand and close the fingers over it firmly (Fig. 190A). Lay the center of a cravat bandage over the upturned wrist. Take the end on the thumb side and bring it up over the back of the hand, opposite the thumb side, and over the two fingers on that side (Fig. 190B). Take the other end and bring it

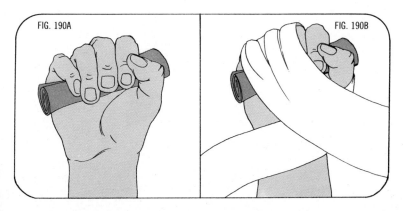

FIG. 190A   FIG. 190B

diagonally across the back of the hand and over the other two fingers (Fig. 190C). The ends should cross over the upturned wrist. Pull down firmly on the crossed ends to hold the fingers tightly against the pad in the palm. Cross the ends in opposite directions around the wrist and tie at the side of the wrist (Fig. 190D).

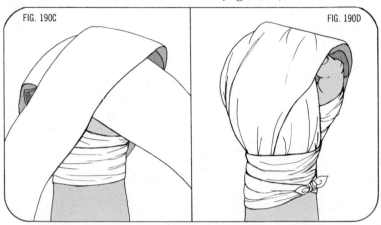

FIG. 190C

FIG. 190D

This dressing should be used only for severe bleeding from wounds of the palm, and only for a short period until bleeding is under control or the victim is seen by a physician. The preferred dressing for wounds of the hand is a bulky compress with fluffs of gauze between the fingers and exposure of all fingertips.

Fingertip Bandage

A series of back-and-forth turns (Fig. 191A), called recurrent turns, are held in place by circular and spiral turns (Figs. 191B,C,

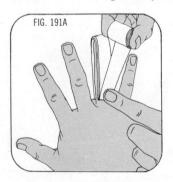

FIG. 191A

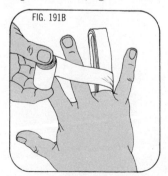

FIG. 191B

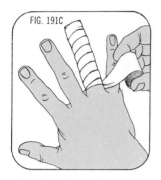 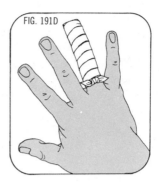

and D). Normally used on fingers, the fingertip bandage may be adapted for use on toes, scalp, or stumps of limbs. When such areas as the scalp are to be covered, the next fold covers the opposite side of the part being covered, and each succeeding fold is worked toward the center until the area is sufficiently covered. This bandage is held in place with circular turns.

Another method of securing the fingertip bandage is to use the figure-of-eight turn to complete its application. From the finger, take the end of the bandage diagonally across the back of the hand to the wrist; encircle one or more times (Fig. 192A). From the opposite side of the wrist, continue by looping at the finger (Fig. 192B). Repeat the figure-of-eight as necessary and tie off at the wrist (Fig. 192C).

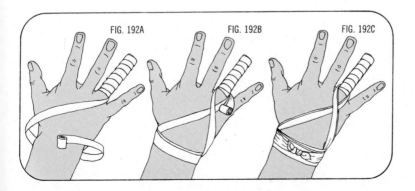

Figure-of-Eight Bandage for Ankle

Anchor the bandage on the instep and take two or three additional turns around the instep. Carry the bandage diagonally upward across the front of the foot, then around the ankle (Figs. 193A and 193B) and diagonally downward across the front of the foot and under the arch. Make several of these figure-of-eight turns, each turn overlapping the previous one by about two-thirds the width of the bandage (Fig. 193C). Occasionally, use an extra turn around the ankle.

Complete by tying off (Fig. 193D).

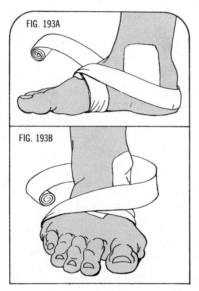

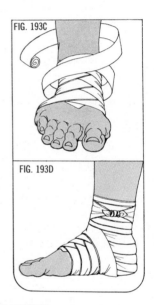

FIRST AID KITS AND SUPPLIES

From your study of first aid you have learned how to improvise a number of bandages, dressings, and splints. It is, of course, more satisfactory to have sterile dressings, prepared splints, and other first aid equipment ready for use before an accident occurs.

There are two general types of first aid kits: (1) the unit type and (2) the cabinet type.

Unit-Type Kits

Unit-type kits have a complete assortment of first aid materials put up in standard packages of unit size or multiples of the unit size and arranged in cases containing 16, 24, or 32 units, with the 16- and the 24-unit kits being the most popular. Each unit package contains one or more individual dressings. Each dressing is complete in itself and is sealed in a sterile wrapper. It contains just enough material to treat a single injury, thus eliminating waste. All liquids are put up in individual, sealed ampules, and consequently cannot deteriorate. There are no bottles to spill or break.

Illustrations and instructions for the use of the contents are on the front of each package. The desired unit packages are easy to locate, because the contents are clearly indicated on the top side in bold type. The unit packages fit like blocks in the case; they cannot shift or become disarranged. These types of kits are probably the most satisfactory for carrying in a car or truck or in a pack.

Standard refills are supplied by various manufacturers and can be changed easily to meet the needs of the purchaser. Unit refills are easy to obtain. The original cost may be slightly higher, but when materials are subject to much handling by many different persons, this type is generally cheaper and more satisfactory in the long run. There is no contamination or waste of unused materials. The kits can be obtained with contents selected to meet the particular needs of the purchaser.

Contents of 16-Unit First Aid Kit

2 units—1″ adhesive compress
2 units—2″ bandage compress
1 unit—3″ bandage compress
1 unit—4″ bandage compress
1 unit—3″ x 3″ plain gauze pads
1 unit—gauze roller bandage
2 units—plain absorbent gauze—1/2 sq. yd.
2 units—plain absorbent gauze—24″ x 72″
3 units—triangular bandages—40″
1 unit—tourniquet, scissors, tweezers

Contents of 24-Unit First Aid Kit

2 units—1″ adhesive compress
2 units—2″ bandage compress
2 units—3″ bandage compress
2 units—4″ bandage compress
1 unit—3″ x 3″ plain gauze pads
2 units—gauze roller bandage

1 unit—eye dressing packet
4 units—plain absorbent gauze—1/2 sq. yd.
3 units—plain absorbent gauze—24" x 72"
4 units—triangular bandages—40"
1 unit—tourniquet, scissors, tweezers

Cabinet-Type Kits

Cabinet kits are made for a wide variety of uses and range in size from pocket versions to large industrial kits. They are made to accept packages in different shapes and sizes. Contents may be varied by the purchaser to suit his particular first aid needs. The extra space in most cabinet kits also allows additional items to be inserted according to user's needs.

Cabinet kits contain a large enough supply of most first aid items to be used for more than a single treatment. However, all sterile materials are individually wrapped.

Cabinet kits carry familiar first aid items that are easily recognized in an emergency. Although the different-size packages allow for some shifting of products in transported kits, they have the advantage of a functional package design that does not waste unnecessary space.

Refills are obtainable from most drugstores or through safety equipment distributors.

Other Kits

Kits can be either purchased or can be assembled from improvised materials. All kits, whether purchased or improvised, are satisfactory if the following points are observed in their selection:

• The kit should be large enough and should have the proper contents for the place where it is to be used.
• The contents should be arranged so that the desired package can be found quickly without unpacking the entire contents.
• Material should be wrapped so that unused portions do not become dirty through handling.

Types and sizes of kits to meet specific needs should be selected and supplied with items recommended by your consulting physician.

15

SUDDEN ILLNESS

First aid workers often encounter emergencies that are not related to injury but arise from either sudden illness or a crisis in a chronic illness. Unless the illness is minor and brief (such as a fainting attack, airsickness, a nosebleed, or a headache), medical assistance should be sought. Although sudden illness is not always urgent, sometimes it endangers a person's life, especially if associated with a heart attack or a massive internal hemorrhage. An important first aid measure in such an instance is to transport the victim to a medical facility as quickly and safely as possible.

ILLNESS EVIDENCED BY UNCONSCIOUSNESS

One of the most puzzling of all emergencies is unconsciousness, because information regarding the sequence of events before the victim collapsed is often limited. Unconsciousness associated with poisoning, asphyxia, head injury, or severe shock has been referred to in previous chapters. In the illnesses described below, unconsciousness varies in both depth and duration.

Fainting

Description

Fainting is a partial or complete loss of consciousness due to temporary insufficiency of blood supply to the brain. It is usually preceded or accompanied by extreme paleness, sweating, coldness of the skin, dizziness, numbness and tingling of the hands and feet, nausea, and sometimes by disturbance of vision; but occasionally a person collapses suddenly without warning.

Recovery of consciousness almost always occurs when the victim falls or is placed in a reclining position, although the fall itself may injure him. The victim should be carefully observed afterward, because fainting might constitute a brief episode in the development of a serious underlying illness.

To prevent a fainting attack, a person who feels weak and dizzy should lie down or bend over with his head at the level of his knees.

First Aid

After a fainting attack has occurred—

- Keep the victim lying down.
- Loosen any tight clothing and keep crowds away.
- If the victim vomits, roll him onto his side or turn his head to the side and, if necessary, wipe out his mouth with your fingers, preferably wrapped in cloth. Hold his chin up to keep his tongue from obstructing his airway.
- Do not pour water over the victim's face, for fear of aspiration; instead, bathe his face gently with cool water.
- Do not give him *any* liquid until he has revived.
- Examine the victim to determine whether he has suffered injury from falling.
- Unless recovery is prompt, seek medical assistance.

Stroke

Description

A stroke, also called "apoplexy" and "cerebrovascular accident," usually involves a spontaneous rupture of a blood vessel in the brain or formation of a clot (thrombus) that interferes with circulation. Strokes usually occur in older people with hardening of the arteries and high blood pressure, but they may also occur in young people as a result of defects in blood vessels of the brain.

Signs and Symptoms

In major strokes, unconsciousness is usual. Other signs and symptoms include—

- Paralysis or weakness on the side of the body opposite the brain lesion, and of facial muscles of either side, according to the part of the brain that is involved.

- Difficulty in breathing and in swallowing.
- Loss of bladder and bowel control.
- Unequal size of the pupils.
- Inability to talk or slurring of speech.

In minor strokes, small blood vessels in the brain are involved. The victim usually does not become unconscious, and the symptoms depend on the location of the hemorrhage and the amount of brain damage. The episode may occur during sleep and be accompanied by headache, confusion, slight dizziness, and other mild complaints. Later, there may be minor difficulties in speech, memory changes, weakness in an arm or leg, or some disturbance in the normal pattern of the personality. When symptoms occur, the first aid worker should advise medical consultation and protect the victim against accident or physical exertion.

First Aid

- Maintain an open airway.
- Position the victim on his side so that secretions will drain from the side of his mouth.
- Do not give him fluids unless he is *fully* conscious and able to swallow. Discontinue fluids if he vomits.
- Call a doctor for medical advice as soon as possible; hospitalization will usually be necessary.

Heart Attack

Description

Heart attack usually involves a clot in one of the blood vessels that supply the heart. It is sometimes called a "coronary"—a short form for "coronary artery thrombosis," "coronary occlusion," or "myocardial infarction"—inasmuch as there is loss of blood supply to a portion of the heart muscle, the myocardium.

Signs and Symptoms

A heart attack may or may not be accompanied by loss of consciousness. If it is severe, the victim may die suddenly. The victim

228 ADVANCED FIRST AID AND EMERGENCY CARE

may have a history of heart disease, or the attack may come with little or no warning. The symptoms and signs include—

- Persistent chest pain, usually under the sternum (breastbone). The pain frequently radiates to one or both shoulders or arms, or the neck or jaw or both.
- Gasping and shortness of breath.
- Extreme pallor or bluish discoloration of the lips, skin, and fingernail beds.
- Extreme prostration.
- Shock (as a rule).
- Swelling of the ankles (which may be an indication of heart disease).

If the pain is in the upper abdomen and is accompanied by nausea and vomiting, the victim may mistakenly think he is having an attack of acute indigestion.

If a heart attack has occurred—

First Aid

- If the victim is not breathing, begin artificial respiration.
- Have someone call for an ambulance equipped with oxygen and have the victim's own doctor notified.
- If the victim has been under medical care, the first-aider should assist in administering prescribed medicine and in carrying out other measures advised by the physician. (Look for some form of emergency medical identification.) If in doubt, confer with the physician by telephone.
- Do not give liquids to an unconscious victim.
- Place the victim in a comfortable position, usually sitting up, and prop him up with pillows, particularly if he is short of breath. His comfort is usually a good guide.

Convulsions and Epilepsy

Convulsions

Description and Causes

A convulsion is an attack of unconsciousness, usually of violent onset, accompanied by rigidity of the muscles of the body, usually lasting from a few seconds to about half a minute and followed by jerking movements, bluish discoloration of the face and lips, foaming at the mouth or drooling, and, finally, gradual subsidence of the paroxysm, after which the victim usually is drowsy or disoriented for a time. During the period of rigidity, the victim may stop breathing, may bite his tongue severely, and may lose bladder and bowel control.

In an infant or small child, a convulsion may occur at the onset of an acute infectious disease, particularly during a period of high fever or severe gastrointestinal illness. Convulsions that develop later in the course of measles, mumps, and other childhood diseases are more serious and might reflect complications of the central nervous system.

Convulsions associated with head injury or brain disease—such as a tumor, an abscess, or hemorrhage—tend to be localized, with rigidity and jerking of groups of muscles, instead of the whole body.

Convulsions can also be caused by eclampsia, a condition that occasionally develops in the late stages of toxemia of pregnancy. Eclampsia can usually be prevented by proper prenatal care. The victim should receive *immediate* hospital treatment.

First Aid

First aid for convulsions should be directed primarily at keeping the victim from hurting himself. If the attack is prolonged and the victim stops breathing, give him mouth-to-mouth or mouth-to-nose resuscitation. (NOTE. Do not place a blunt object between the victim's teeth. Do not restrain him or pour any liquid into his mouth. Do not place a child in a tub of water.) If repeated convulsions occur, call for medical help immediately or take the victim to a hospital.

Epilepsy

Description

Epilepsy is a chronic disease, usually of unknown cause, usually characterized by repeated convulsions ("grand mal seizures"), often preceded by a warning sensation known as an "aura." The victim may be able to lie down quickly, or his family may be able to tell that an attack is beginning by the sudden paleness of his face or by his behavior. Mouth-to-nose resuscitation may be the only effective way to ventilate a victim of grand mal seizure if his mouth is tightly closed owing to contraction. From 15 to 20 percent of victims develop flap valve obstruction of exhalation by the soft palate, and because of this high incidence of expiratory obstruction created by the soft palate, mouth-to-nose ventilation must be accomplished in a way that leaves the mouth open for exhalation. If the teeth cannot be separated, the lips should be parted to permit passive exhalation. Much research has been carried out on epilepsy in recent years, and excellent preventive treatment is available; for this reason, physicians should determine the type and cause of every episode of convulsion.

A milder form of epilepsy, characterized by "petit mal seizures," occurs *without convulsions*. There may be only brief twitching of muscles and momentary loss of awareness of the surroundings; the victim may be seen staring fixedly at an object or off into the distance. This type of disturbance is less common than that which produces grand mal seizures. Diagnoses of both forms of epilepsy are made by brain wave tracings.

First Aid

First aid for epilepsy is the same as for other convulsions, with primary effort being made to keep the victim from hurting himself. After a seizure, the victim should be allowed to sleep or rest.

Acute Alcoholism

Unconsciousness may be a complication of acute intoxication from alcoholic beverages; but the odor of alcohol on a person's breath, without other evidence of overindulgence, does not necessarily mean that he is intoxicated. In the absence of other information, special tests can determine whether enough alochol has been consumed to cause unconsciousness.

The signs and symptoms of alcohol intoxication and first aid procedures are covered in chapter 8.

Crises Related to Diabetes

Hyperglycemia

Hyperglycemia—too much sugar in the blood—is generally associated with unconsciousness only in diabetic coma, which may occur in a diabetic who has had inadequate treatment. He may not even know that he has diabetes. Such conditions as infection or injury in a diabetic may lead to diabetic coma, but the unconsciousness, as a rule, does not come on suddenly. The person is likely to be drowsy and confused for some time. His breathing becomes deep and rapid, and his breath has a peculiar fruity odor. If the diabetic has been under treatment, he often will have a card in his wallet or a medical identification tag stating that he is a diabetic; or relatives, acquaintances, or medications at hand may indicate the cause of coma.

There is no adequate first aid treatment for hyperglycemia or diabetic coma; *immediate hospital treatment is necessary.*

Hypoglycemia

Description and Causes

Hypoglycemia (commonly called "insulin reaction" or "insulin shock")—too little sugar in the blood—may be caused by an overdose of insulin in a diabetic patient, failure to obtain food after taking medication (which lowers the concentration of sugar in the blood), unusual exercise, or emotional factors. Patients with mild diabetes seldom have this problem. However, diabetic children are particularly prone to insulin shock.

Hypoglycemia is also related to conditions other than those associated with diabetes; for example, a young person with unstable regulation of blood sugar may experience hypoglycemia after skipping a meal or in midmorning or midafternoon. Fainting is particularly likely when energy has been expended in vigorous exercise or in association with emotional stress.

Signs and Symptoms

Fainting from hypoglycemia is commonly preceded by hunger, a gnawing sensation in the stomach, weakness, dizziness, a jittery feeling, a cold sweat, paleness, tremor of the hands, and dimness of vision. But hypoglycemia may also develop *without* warning. This occurrence is particularly dangerous when the victim is driving an automobile or in circumstances such as athletic activity, when he may injure himself, perhaps by falling, or when swimming alone.

First Aid

First aid treatment for hypoglycemia is to raise the victim's blood sugar concentration as quickly as possible. If there are preliminary symptoms, any food will do; but candy, soft drinks, sugar, fruit juice, or anything else sweet is most effective and may prevent unconsciousness. Remember that coffee and tea have no food value in themselves; sugar must be added. A diabetic, or any other person with a history of attacks of hypoglycemia, should carry hard candy with him and eat one or two pieces every hour or two *in advance* of strenuous exercise or while driving a car. The first-aider will usually find that at the beginning of an attack of hypoglycemia the victim will be able to cooperate by swallowing candy or a sugar-sweetened soft drink—one small sip (or even one or two drops) at a time. Seek medical assistance if the victim does not respond readily.

Hypoglycemia with unconsciousness is an extremely urgent medical emergency. The rescuer should move the victim with all reasonable speed to a nearby medical facility, which should be alerted to expect arrival of the victim. Prior notification is useful so that 50

percent dextrose or glucagon can be immediately available at the
time of the victim's arrival.

HEMORRHAGE

Internal bleeding related to injury is discussed in chapter 2. Hemorrhage from the various organs into the body cavities with or without injury constitutes an emergency.

Description, Signs, and Symptoms

Internal hemorrhage sometimes has no immediate outward indication. After a sudden massive hemorrhage—for example, from a bleeding ulcer of the stomach—the victim may simply collapse in shock. There will be extreme paleness, rapid pulse, and perhaps tenderness over the affected area. Often there will be a history of chronic disturbance of digestion, pain after eating, or other symptoms, depending on the source of internal bleeding.

If fresh blood is brought up from the lungs or vomited, it may be impossible to determine the origin of the hemorrhage, because blood from the lungs may be swallowed first and then vomited. This condition also occurs occasionally with severe nosebleed. If there is pink-tinged, foamy sputum, it is from the lungs. Vomitus the color of coffee grounds indicates that old blood from a previous hemorrhage is present in the stomach or upper intestinal tract. A very large amount of blood may be brought up by retching and vomiting in cases of chronic liver disease, in which the blood vessels in the lower end of the esophagus have enlarged and ruptured, owing to increased pressure and their thin walls.

The stools may contain streaks of blood from hemorrhoids or from a rectal crack or fissure; such bleeding in small amounts is not ordinarily cause for alarm. A considerable amount of bright red blood in the stools indicates hemorrhage from the lower bowel. Blood from the upper regions of the colon and small intestine will usually give the stools a tarry appearance—like the stools after a person has taken tonics, some vitamin mixtures, or drugs containing iron.

Bleeding from the bladder, kidneys, or urethra may give the urine a smoky appearance; bright red blood may be seen in the urine when there is acute bleeding or infection or after an injury.

Unusually severe vaginal bleeding may be related to menstrual periods or may occur after menopause. One of the commonest causes is a miscarriage during the early weeks of pregnancy—often before pregnancy has even been diagnosed. These conditions require immediate medical consultation and treatment, as do all instances of abnormal bleeding during pregnancy or after childbirth. A ruptured tubal pregnancy is a critical emergency condition because of internal bleeding.

First Aid

Always consider the possibility of massive internal bleeding when there is sudden collapse, marked paleness, rapid and weak pulse, thirst, restlessness, anxiety, rapid breathing, and shock. First aid in such cases consists of gentle handling of the victim, checking of the airway, keeping the victim lying down, summoning medical help by telephone, and arranging for immediate transportation to the hospital. Oxygen should be given on the way if available.

When there is hemorrhage from the lungs or stomach, have the victim sit up and lean forward, if possible; or place him on his side or abdomen with his head to the side and slightly lowered and hold his jaw forward to keep his airway open. If you have a suction bulb, use it to clear the back of his throat; otherwise, wipe out his mouth often with a cloth. Above all, do *not* give the victim anything by mouth.

The first-aider will rarely encounter a person who has tendencies toward excessive or prolonged bleeding on slight injury owing to defects in the clotting mechanism of the victim's blood. Such a person will probably have a personal or family history of the disorder (hemophilia) and should be taken to a hospital for treatment whenever bleeding cannot be relieved.

PAIN

Severe pain, alone or in combination with other symptoms, is always distressing to the victim and to his family. It is often difficult for an onlooker to distinguish pain from fear, anxiety, or panic. Therefore, every effort should be made to relieve anxiety by assuming a calm manner, whether or not you feel calm; by frequent reassurance; by gentle handling; and by removal of such irritants as lights in the victim's eyes and loud noises. If there is pain without injury, try to find out how and when the pain started, the exact location, the kind of pain (such as dull, sharp, cramping, or burning), and other symptoms, in order to relay this information over the telephone to a physician, if necessary.

Headache

The most severe headaches are those accompanying head injury, cerebral hemorrhage, and brain disease. Migraine headaches are fairly common, as are those related to acute sinusitis. Headaches often occur in women during the premenstrual period, when fluid may collect in all the tissues of the body as a result of salt accumulation. Headaches may be associated with eyestrain and a variety of other conditions, including onset of an acute infectious disease in which fever and generalized aching are common. The headache may be due to tension and can be relieved by household pain-relieving remedies such as aspirin, rest, cold applications, or relaxation. Anyone whose headaches are unusually severe or frequent should be examined by a physician.

Pain in the Eyes

Emergency treatment is required when a sudden, sharp pain develops in the eyes, accompanied by dimness of vision, halos around lights, or other complaints that might indicate onset of glaucoma, a disease characterized by increased pressure inside the eyeball. Marked impairment, or even loss, of vision may result within as short a period as a few hours. Medical attention must be sought *immediately*. All older persons should have their eyes checked periodically for increased pressure.

The increasing use of contact lenses in recent years has resulted in more eye injuries as the lenses are inserted or removed or when they are left in too long. A person who wears contact lenses should carry a note to that effect so that in case of injury or prolonged unconsciousness, and if medical care is not available within several hours, proper removal of the lenses will prevent corneal damage. The first-aider should wash his hands carefully before removing the victim's lens, if possible. The preferred method is to hold both eyelids open with your fingers and flush the eye with a gentle stream of clean water from any source (Fig. 194A). This action should loosen the contact lens and flush it away. If this procedure fails, gently slide the lens off the cornea to the side (Fig. 194B and 194C). Then, under strong light, lift off the lens, taking care not to scratch the eyeball with your fingernail (Fig. 194D). *Do not lose the lens.* If you cannot remove the lens, it may be left on the eyeball until the lens is removed by a physician, as long as it does not rest on the cornea.

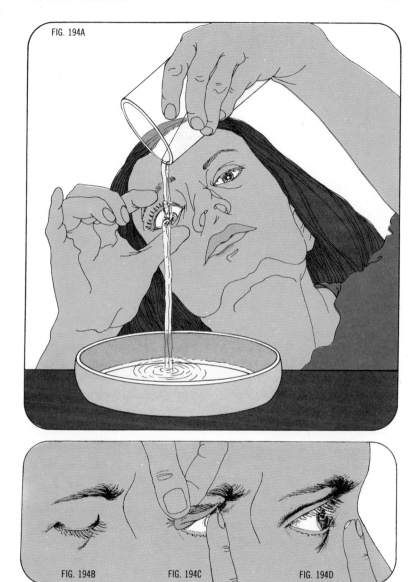

FIG. 194A

FIG. 194B   FIG. 194C   FIG. 194D

Pain in the Ears

An acute earache may be extremely painful and may end with spontaneous rupture of the eardrum, whether caused by increased pressure or by a middle ear infection. During air travel, as the air pressure changes in takeoff and landing, pressure within the eustachian tube (which connects the throat with the middle ear) may be equalized by chewing gum, swallowing, or yawning. If these measures are not sufficient to relieve pain, deafness, and the stopped-up feeling, take in a deep breath, hold it, and, with nostrils pinched together, blow forcibly for a few seconds before actually exhaling. Do not place any medication in the ear canal after rupture of an eardrum, whether or not drainage is apparent. In a simple earache, if fever is present or if pain is unrelieved after a few hours either by heat applied externally or by home medication, a physician should be consulted.

Toothache

Causes

A toothache may be related to a deep cavity in a tooth or to infection at the root.

First Aid

First aid consists of cleansing the mouth, inserting a small bit of cotton into the cavity to exclude air (oil of cloves on the cotton is a time-honored local anesthetic in such cases), applying either a hot or cold compress (whichever gives the most relief), and using simple household remedies for pain.

Chest Pain

Description, Signs, and Symptoms

The two most common emergencies associated with heart disease are *angina pectoris* (the Latin term for pain in the chest) and *coronary thrombosis*. Coronary thrombosis is discussed on page 227 as a cause of unconsciousness and, at times, of temporary cardiac arrest or of sudden death. The pain in both these conditions is essentially the same, in that it is "vicelike." It persists for a long period in coronary thrombosis, but typically for only a few minutes (or even seconds) in angina. Many persons have repeated attacks of angina over a period of years and carry nitroglycerine tablets or amyl nitrite ampules with them.

The pain in angina and coronary thrombosis is in the chest underneath the sternum. (Sometimes it also involves the upper abdomen, the neck, or the left arm.) There is a feeling of impending death, and the victim of the attack usually becomes extremely still. His breathing is shallow. His face is extremely pale or bluish, and he may be covered with sweat. He is in shock and should be handled gently. Artificial respiration may be appropriate, and even life-saving, in some instances. In angina, the victim usually recovers quickly, whereas coronary thrombosis requires prolonged treatment, hospitalization, and convalescence.

Chest pain that is not associated with heart disease occurs often. It may be due to *lung disease*, such as pneumonia or bronchitis, or to pain in the muscle fibers of the chest wall. *Shingles* (herpes zoster) is characterized by a very severe burning pain that follows the course of a spinal nerve; when it occurs in the chest wall it may be confused with heart attack.

First Aid

First aid measures consist of giving the victim nitroglycerine or amyl nitrite for angina, if he has his own medication. The taking of these drugs should be avoided if coronary thrombosis is suspected. Prop the victim up for easier breathing, if he desires. Send for an ambulance with an oxygen supply if relief of pain or shortness of breath is not obtained within a few minutes. An irregular pulse is an ominous sign: medical attention should be sought without delay.

Abdominal Pain

All abdominal pain should be investigated—especially unusual pain that comes on rather suddenly, is accompanied by fever, and is not characterized by repeated attacks of diarrhea (although vomiting and diarrhea may occur at the beginning of almost any abdominal crisis).

Persons who have had abdominal surgery may experience abdominal pain as a result of obstruction from adhesions and should be examined promptly.

Food Poisoning

The most common source of acute abdominal pain is probably food poisoning, which usually results from swallowing food that contains bacterial toxins, even if bacteria in the food have been killed by reheating. (For chemical poisons in plants and fish, see chapter 7.) Food poisoning may be seen in epidemic form if a family or a large group of persons have eaten protein-containing foods, such as chicken salad, creamed dishes, custard, canned meats, or any other preparations with milk, eggs, or meat that have been inadequately refrigerated, have stood too long, or have been contaminated by a food handler who has a cold, a boil on his skin, or other infection.

Allergic Reactions to Food

Allergic reactions to food at times resemble symptoms of food poisoning. There is often a history of previous attacks (when the victim has eaten specific foods, such as seafood or strawberries). A skin rash is also a symptom. A specific type of food poisoning, and a particularly lethal one, is *botulism,* caused most commonly by contamination of home-canned beans and corn and occasionally by commercial products. An effective antitoxin has been prepared for use in cases of botulism. Although it may not be available in time to save victims of the most severe cases, it may be given to persons who have eaten foods suspected of being contaminated but who have not yet developed symptoms.

If an attack of vomiting or diarrhea is unusually severe or persists more than a few hours, a physician should be consulted. Meanwhile, if vomiting subsides in a short period, or does not occur at all, such liquids as hot tea or carbonated drinks should be given cautiously, in sips, to replace some of the fluids that have been lost and thus prevent dehydration. Solid food should be withheld until the attack is over, approximately 24 hours. The victim should stay in bed.

If there is any question about whether a person has been poisoned by drugs or chemicals, seek medical aid as quickly as possible. Do *not* give laxative drugs to any person with abdominal pain.

Acute Appendicitis

Acute appendicitis may occur at any age. It is generally characterized by the onset of pain in the upper midabdomen, later shifting to the lower right side, with considerable tenderness in that area. Slight fever may be present. Because delay increases the danger of rupture of the appendix, medical attention should be obtained immediately. Even if symptoms subside, medical advice should be sought, because the appendix may be dangerously diseased, even if the pain subsides. Meanwhile, do not give a laxative; withhold food and water; and do not apply heat to abdomen.

Hernia

Hernia (rupture) is a protrusion, or bulging, in a weak area of the abdominal wall, caused by a loop of the bowel pushing through or against the abdominal wall. Hernia may also appear in the scar of an abdominal operation, at the navel, or just below the midgroin. It is more common in obese persons, but it may affect the strong or the weak, the young or the old. During the first weeks the rupture may cause some pain; later, less discomfort. The bulge generally disappears when the victim lies down and reappears when he rises. In time, it may increase in size; if it does, surgery will probably be recommended by the physician. There is a danger that a hernia may become "strangulated" and that constriction effects may shut off the blood supply of the loop of bowel, necessitating an emergency operation because the bowel part cannot survive long without blood.

When a rupture is first noted, the victim should refrain from heavy lifting and vigorous activity and should seek medical attention. Do not press on the bulge to force it inward, because its path is seldom straight and the pressure may damage the bowel. If the bulge persists when the victim lies down and the bowel loop appears to be caught in the hernia, the knee-chest position may be tried (Fig. 195):

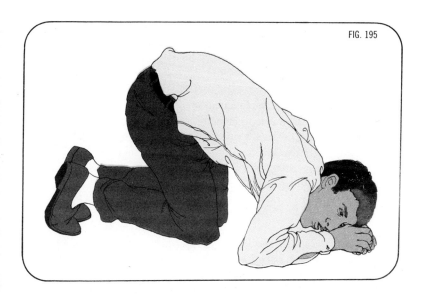

FIG. 195

The victim lies on his abdomen and then brings his knees up under his chest so that his buttocks are raised high. If this effort also fails,

he should lie on his back with a pillow under his knees and be taken
for medical examination.

Gallstones and Kidney Stones

Gallstones and kidney stones can cause excruciating pain in the
abdomen if a gallstone blocks the bile duct or a kidney stone blocks
the ureter (the tube from the kidney to the bladder). The pain is
colicky; that is, there is a paroxysm of severe pain, followed by slight
relief, and then repetition of the pain. Immediate treatment may not
be necessary, but the victim usually will require advice and treatment by a physician.

Perforation of an Ulcer

Perforation of an ulcer in the stomach or elsewhere in the gastrointestinal tract is usually accompanied by intense pain, tenderness, and shock. The victim should be taken to a hospital immediately. Do not give him anything by mouth and do not apply either
warm or cold compresses to his abdomen.

Neck Pain

Spasm of the neck muscles, commonly called a "crick in the
neck," is often a source of acute discomfort. If it fails to respond to
hot applications and home remedies for pain, a physician should be
consulted. The condition is urgent if neck pain is accompanied by
marked rigidity of the muscles so that the neck cannot be bent
forward. (The muscles of the neck and back may even be arched
backward. This condition is usually an indication that the central
nervous system is involved, owing to an infection, such as a childhood contagious disease, acute poliomyelitis, meningitis, or brain
hemorrhage.) Rigidity of the neck muscles should be cause for alarm;
a physician should be consulted immediately.

Back Pain

Acute back pain may result from spasm of the lumbar muscles. In
a person who has had repeated difficulty, this pain is often the result
of injury—perhaps even a slight, unnoticed injury.

Stiffness, pain with or without motion, chronic aching, and some
disability of function accompany the noncrippling kind of rheuma-
tism or arthritis, which is common in middle-aged and older persons.

Pains tend to shift from joint to joint. Temporary relief may be obtained by home medication and by application of heat (in the form of hot packs, warm baths, or liniments). Emergency treatment is rarely required.

Rectal Pain

Description and Causes

The pain from a thrombosed hemorrhoid (or "piles") and other types of rectal disorders, such as an abscess or a malignant or benign tumor, may be extremely severe, because it is often related to a spasm of the muscles in the area.

First Aid

Sitting in a tub of warm water or applying heat and steady pressure on the perineal muscles may provide some relief, along with taking medication for pain and using a soothing suppository, if available. Medical consultation may be required. Persistent or recurring rectal pain should always be investigated because of the danger of cancer.

Acute Retention of Urine

Description and Causes

Inability to pass urine may be a complication of injury, disease, surgery, or childbirth. It may also occur as the result of exposure to cold or other conditions. Enlargement of the prostate is a common cause in men in the older age group. The victim may complain of severe pain and distress, and his bladder may be felt as a large mass in the lower abdomen.

First Aid

In many instances, it is necessary to have a physician insert a soft rubber catheter into the bladder to permit passage of urine, but first aid measures should be tried first. These include application of warm (not hot), moist packs over the lower abdomen or a warm sitz bath. Running of water in the room or pouring warm water over the genitalia may be effective, by suggestion. If relief of retention is not obtained, consult a physician or have the victim go to a hospital for catheterization.

Pelvic Pain

Pelvic pain is often incapacitating in menstrual disorders but rarely constitutes an emergency. Sudden pain in the lower abdomen on either side may occur with tubal infections and tubal pregnancy, in which case a physician should be consulted immediately. A physician should also be consulted immediately for any acute upper or lower abdominal pain during normal pregnancy, because any type of abdominal emergency, such as appendicitis or acute gall bladder attack, may occur during pregnancy. For *dysmenorrhea* (painful menstruation) that does not respond to mild medication for pain, to heat, and to bed rest, a physician should be consulted.

Leg Pain

Acute, severe, cramping pain in the legs may occur during exercise or at rest. Night cramps are particularly common but usually do not constitute an emergency. Massage, stretching of the cramping muscles, and local heat may be sufficient to give relief. Cramping that is related to exercise and that subsides with rest is sometimes a symptom of circulatory difficulty in the legs. A physician should be consulted.

Pain Associated With Infection

Acute, throbbing pain almost always accompanies localized infection, regardless of the kind or location (see chapter 2). A common local infection is the boil, which affects the hair follicles of the skin or the eyelid. Symptoms and first aid are the same as for infections that follow injury (see page 40).

Difficulty in Breathing

Difficulties in breathing associated with injury, asphyxia, choking, and other conditions are discussed in chapter 5.

Chronic Heart Disease

Persons with chronic heart disease typically wake up in the night extremely short of breath and gasping for air. Coughing may produce frothy, pink-tinged sputum. In mild cases, sitting upright in bed or in a chair will relieve the symptoms. Otherwise, medical assistance should be obtained. The attack may be a warning of coronary thrombosis (see page 227).

Croup

Description

Another type of breathing difficulty, particularly common in small children, is croup, a type of acute laryngitis characterized by marked spasm of the larynx with a ringing, metallic cough and great difficulty in inhaling, so that the respiratory muscles of the chest are pulled in tightly, as in other types of obstruction of the larynx.

First Aid

The spasm will often subside quickly if the child is exposed to moist heat. Take him into the bathroom and turn on all the hot water faucets, especially in the shower. A steam kettle can also be used, with a paper cone attached to the spout; or a croup tent may be improvised. In every instance of croup, diptheria should be considered, unless the child has had adequate immunization. If relief is not obtained by the measures described above and the spasm of the larynx is becoming more severe, wrap the child in a blanket, forming a tent over his face so that he will not breathe in cold air, and take him to a hospital emergency room. Have someone call ahead to a physician or to the hospital.

Asthma and Asthmatic Bronchitis

Signs and Symptoms

Acute asthma or an attack of acute asthmatic bronchitis often precipitates wheezing in the chest and marked difficulty in breathing. The victim is usually known to have an allergy and often has medication on hand.

First Aid

First aid consists of administering an antihistamine drug if one has been prescribed by the victim's physician; propping the victim up; and providing warm, moist air if spasm of the larynx develops. A flare-up of acute asthma or asthmatic bronchitis is often related to a respiratory infection, and an attack may be so severe in a child that immediate hospital care is necessary.

Hiccups

Description

Hiccups, due to a spasm of the diaphragm, are rarely severe enough to interfere with breathing or to require medical aid.

First Aid

Holding the breath, breathing in and out of a paper bag to increase the carbon dioxide concentration in the blood, drinking a glass of warm water slowly, or applying a cold pack to the abdomen are successful first aid remedies in most cases. If hiccups persist for a long time, call a physician.

Anaphylaxis

Description and Causes

Anaphylaxis (anaphylactic shock) is a very serious, acute, allergic reaction of the body to overwhelming sensitization by a foreign protein. It may be produced when a susceptible person is stung by a bee, has eaten particular foods, has had an injection of horse serum or some drugs (for example, penicillin). The victim becomes weak and pale and collapses. He has great difficulty in breathing, complains of severe chest pain, and may have convulsions. Death can result within minutes.

First Aid

The first-aider should summon medical aid as quickly as possible. Administer artificial respiration, if it is warranted. An anthihistamine tablet should be given, if available. (A person who has severe allergies or who reacts violently to bee or wasp stings should consult his physician for proper advice and preventive medication. If an antihistamine has been prescribed it should be given to the victim without delay).

RAPID HEARTBEAT

An episode of rapid heartbeat or palpitation may be cause for alarm on the part of the victim. Usually, the person becomes "heart-conscious" because of occasional irregular beats, but these are common, especially in older people. Such an irregular beat ordinarily comes a little early in the heartbeat cycle and is followed by a slightly longer pause than usual. This occurrence is interpreted as a "skipped" or "missed" beat and is usually noticed when the person is lying down and is quiet. Actually, no beats are missed. Although this condition is not uncommon in healthy persons, persistent episodes call for medical attention. Often, the frightened person begins to breathe deeply and may hyperventilate.

Rapid heartbeat normally is related to increased exertion and strong emotion, and a person may be frightened by the increase in the strength of the pulsations that are felt and easily seen. Mild sedation may be appropriate in this type of rapid heartbeat and also in a fairly common condition called "paroxysmal tachycardia" (rapid heartbeat). Paroxysmal tachycardia is characterized by extreme rapidity of the pulse that comes on suddenly and reverts to normal just as suddenly. The pulse may be too fast to count, and the victim may become faint, weak, and breathless. This condition is a disturbance of function, often related to smoking or to excessive intake of caffeine in coffee or soft drinks. If attacks occur often, medication may be used to stop them quickly or prevent recurrence. The attacks are usually so short that the heart rate returns to normal before medication can take effect. Medical diagnosis is usually made on the basis of the history.

HIGH FEVER

Extremely high body temperature constitutes an emergency. In general, children tend to have higher temperatures than adults. Medical advice should be obtained whenever a person's temperature stays at 102°F or over for more than a few minutes. Hospitalization is usually recommended, except for transient high fever at the onset of a childhood disease. A second rise in temperature later may be a warning of complications that require specific treatment.

MENTAL AND EMOTIONAL DISTURBANCES

The most important emotional disturbances in persons who are fairly well adjusted are acute anxiety, grief or depression, and panic (which is a reaction to intense fear that may lead to disorganized behavior). All three may be helped by reassurance and by keeping the affected person distracted and busy. If the person becomes greatly disturbed, a physician should be consulted or, in an acute emergency, the police or an ambulance crew should be called. Do not restrain the person unless it is absolutely necessary, and do not argue with him. Distraction is of more value, especially if you are afraid he may harm himself.

If the victim of a sudden, severe, emotional disturbance is not a member of your own family, try to have a witness at hand. The relatives of a mental patient being treated in his home should have received previous instruction in the administration of medications and in the handling of crises, such as violent outbursts of temper and severe depression. They should find out, also, whether medications that are dangerous when combined with alcoholic beverages have been taken (see chapter 7).

Some signs of mental illness are—
- Hallucinations (seeing things or hearing sounds that are nonexistent).
- Ideas of persecution.
- Marked and persistent insomnia (inability to sleep).
- Withdrawal from normal activities.
- Spells of weeping.
- Threats of suicide.
- Persistent temper outbursts.
- Excessive drinking.
- Signs of addiction to any drugs (especially multiple marks on the skin made from hypodermic injections); repeated use of drugs that produce hallucinations (see chapter 8).
- Unfounded physical complaints.
- Crime or serious juvenile delinquency.
- Carelessness in dress in a person previously well groomed.

In elderly people, personality changes and mental illness may result from small, unnoticed strokes or other organic changes.

Any person who is severely depressed or who threatens suicide should have constant companionship until the crisis has passed, and all harmful implements and drugs should be locked in an inaccessible place. Any threat of suicide should be taken seriously. Seek medical consultation.

For emotional problems related to the strains and stresses of everyday living, ventilation, or airing out, of feelings with sympathetic listeners (including clergymen, social workers, and trained personnel in mental health associations and service agencies) is helpful both for the disturbed person and for members of his immediate family.

16

EMERGENCY CHILDBIRTH

Although pregnancy and labor are usually normal physiologic processes, the health and safety of both mother and child may depend on regular visits to a physician for prenatal care and on medical assistance at the time of delivery. At times, complications arise that lead to emergency situations. Three of these have been mentioned previously: a ruptured tubal pregnancy with concealed hemorrhage into the abdominal cavity, unusual bleeding from the vagina at any stage, and convulsions associated with pregnancy—that is, eclampsia.

The onset of labor is usually gradual, and there is sufficient time for consultation with a physician by telephone and for transportation to a hospital for delivery of an infant under sterile conditions. Nowadays in the United States, 95 percent of all infants are born in hospitals, and the births of 98 percent are attended by physicians. Having proper medical care is the best way to have a baby, for the safety of mother and child. The procedures described below are not substitutes for medical care before, during, and after birth but are given because the first aid worker may at times be called on to assist in emergency childbirth. If birth is imminent, every effort should be made to seek medical help or to find a relative or neighbor who has assisted in childbirth. In every instance in which emergency childbirth occurs outside the hospital, the mother and infant should be taken to a hospital as soon as possible for examination and treatment.

SIGNS AND SYMPTOMS OF IMPENDING CHILDBIRTH

A woman having her first child, as well as one who has had several previous pregnancies, may experience a very rapid course of labor. Because of miscalculations in the anticipated delivery date, premature onset of labor after an accident, delay in transportation, and other such factors, a woman's labor may begin unexpectedly. If the labor contractions are approximately 2 minutes apart, and the woman is straining or pushing down with contractions, crying out constantly, and perhaps warning that the baby is coming, she needs help immediately.

DELIVERY PROCEDURES

Position of the Patient

Underclothing that will interfere with delivery should be removed as quickly as possible or pushed up out of the way, and the woman should lie down on her back, with knees bent, feet flat, and thighs separated widely (Figs. 196A and 196B)—on the floor, the seat of an

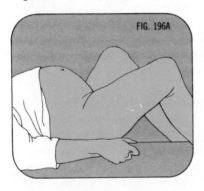
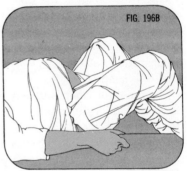

FIG. 196A   FIG. 196B

automobile, the ground, or any other flat surface. If the woman is at home and there is time, she may lie across a bed in the same position, with her feet resting on two straight chairs and her thighs and abdomen covered with clean towels or sheets. In a public place, if others are around, quickly arrange for as much privacy as possible by having people stand around the woman with their backs turned to her to shield the scene from others.

Place newspapers, a clean cloth, or clothing under the woman's buttocks, if any such material is available. If water is close by, wash your hands.

Inspection of the Presenting Part

Inspect the opening of the woman's birth canal (vagina) to determine whether the baby's head is visible at the time of contractions.

(It recedes back up into the canal between contractions.) The back of its head is usually the presenting part; a wrinkled scalp and hair may be noted, although the head may still be enclosed in the bag of waters. If the woman has had previous pregnancies, and the exposed area of the baby's head is approximately the size of a 50-cent piece, or larger, delivery will probably occur within a few minutes, during the next two or three contractions. If the woman is having her first child and the exposed area of the baby's head is smaller than a 50-cent piece, proceed to the nearest hospital, if it is not more than 20 minutes away. You will probably arrive in time. Meanwhile, encourage the woman not to bear down or strain with contractions, but instead to breathe in and out rapidly with short, panting breaths.

Never try to hold back the baby's head or tell the woman to cross her legs to delay delivery. Such maneuvers may seriously injure the infant. Never place your hands or fingers into the birth canal at any time, because of the danger of infection. Allow the delivery to proceed without interference until the baby's head has emerged fully.

A rare but urgent crisis exists when, upon rupture of the bag of waters, the cord protrudes into the birth canal. The patient should be taken to the hospital *immediately* and meanwhile should *stay* in a jackknife or knee-chest position to relieve pressure on the cord and prevent shutting off the blood supply to the infant.

Delivery of the Head

As the infant's head emerges, be prepared to guide and support it with your hands to prevent its becoming contaminated with blood, mucus, and fecal material. If the bag of waters breaks at this point, birth will probably take place rapidly. If the baby's head passes through the birth canal to the outside with the bag still unbroken, tear it with your fingers to let the fluid escape and prevent aspiration as the infant takes its first breaths. As a rule, the infant's face is down (Figs. 197A through 197C); positions with the face up are much less common.

When the head emerges, check it once to see whether the umbilical cord—which looks like a soft, thick, gelatinous white rope—is wrapped around the infant's neck. If so, gently but quickly slip it over the baby's head with your forefinger between its neck and the cord. If the cord is wrapped around its neck more than once, or for some other reason you cannot slip it over the baby's head, it must be cut immediately to prevent strangulation. Squeeze the cut ends with gauze, cloth, or your fingers until ties can be applied. (See below.)

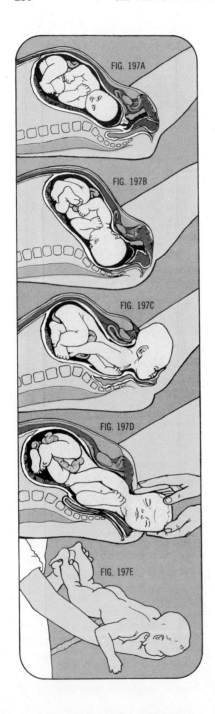

FIG. 197A

FIG. 197B

FIG. 197C

FIG. 197D

FIG. 197E

If any part of the baby other than its head is seen at the opening of the birth canal—for example, its buttocks (a breech birth), hand, or foot—the chances for a safe birth are much less, and you should proceed at once to the nearest hospital. Do not pull on any part and do not attempt to deliver the infant yourself.

As the baby's head emerges, it turns naturally to one side. Do not turn it. Hold it gently, and as soon as possible, wipe out the infant's mouth with clean cloth, gauze, or facial tissues. Do not pull on its head.

Delivery of the Shoulders

As soon as the baby's shoulders start through the birth canal, lift slightly upward with your hands, supporting its head and neck, to assist them to emerge (Fig. 197D). The rest of its body will be expelled quickly (Fig. 197E). Remember that a baby is slippery.

Resuscitation of the Infant

The most important <u>first aid</u> procedure in emergency childbirth is assisting the infant to begin breathing. First, keep it warm. It may be dark blue; but within 1 or 2 minutes, when it starts breathing and crying, it will gradually turn a rosy pink. To assist it, lower its head, elevating the feet and the lower part of the body by grasping the ankles with your hand (protected by a clean cloth if possible, to prevent slipping). Stroke along the baby's neck from its chest toward its mouth with a milking motion, and wipe out its mouth again. If the infant is not crying, rub its back or flick the bottom of its feet with your thumb and forefinger. If it is still not breathing, give artificial respiration in gentle puffs, through the mouth and nose, one every 5 seconds. As soon as it is breathing well, wrap it up, if possible, and put it down with its head extended back and a pad under its shoulders to keep the airway open. If the mother can help, she may hold the baby on her abdomen. Watch the cord—it should be kept slack, without any tension.

Cutting the Cord

No harm will result if the infant is left attached to the afterbirth by the umbilical cord until the mother can be taken to the hospital. This procedure is preferable to cutting the cord with unclean instruments or using an improper cord tie. If the cord is strangling the baby as its head emerges, however, the cord *must* be cut as a life-saving procedure.

If the decision is made to tie and cut the cord while waiting for contractions to resume to expel the placenta, wait until all pulsations of the cord have stopped—about 5 minutes. At home, use a *new* razor blade (one-edged, if possible) or take the time to boil scissors or soak them in rubbing alcohol (or after-shave lotion or other alcohol-based preparations) for 20 minutes. Boil new white shoelaces or narrow strips of clean white cloth for 20 minutes; they may be applied wet. (Sterile cord ties may be purchased or prepared in advance by sterilization in aluminum foil in an oven at 350° F for 3 hours.)

The cord *must not be cut closer than 4 inches from the infant's navel.* Tie a square knot (or two or three simple knots) 4 to 6 inches from the baby and a second knot 8 inches from the baby (Fig. 198). Cut between. (The cord end attached to the baby dries out, shrivels up, and falls off within a few days.)

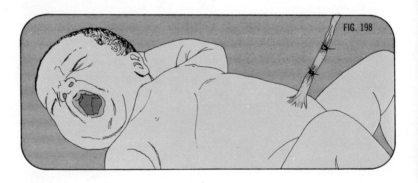

FIG. 198

Expulsion of the Afterbirth

Shortly after the birth of the baby, the mother's contractions resume in preparation for expelling the afterbirth (placenta), as it detaches from the wall of the womb (uterus). Do not pull on the cord, and do not push hard on the mother's abdomen in an effort to hurry things along. Severe damage to the uterus may result, with perhaps fatal hemorrhage. As soon as the afterbirth emerges, however, place your hand over the mother's lower abdomen and *massage* the uterus gently but firmly for a few minutes. The massaging will stimulate the uterus to contract and will help control bleeding. Repeat every 5 minutes for at least the next hour or until the mother is seen by a physician. Save the afterbirth and take it to the hospital with you.

CARE AFTER DELIVERY

After a home delivery, gently cleanse the vaginal opening with a clean, moist towel, or pour soapy water over the vaginal opening, from above toward the rectum, and rinse by pouring warm water over the entire area. Lay a sanitary napkin or other suitable clean cotton material across the vaginal opening.

Give the mother tea, coffee, or other fluids and keep her warm. Do not attempt to cleanse the infant of the white, greasy protective coating covering its skin. Do not wash its eyes, ears, or nose. Check to be sure that its breathing is normal and that it is kept warm during transfer to the hospital.

If the afterbirth is not expelled within a reasonable length of time or if it is not completely expelled, there is danger of hemorrhage. Medical care should be sought without delay. Do not pull on the afterbirth or on the cord.

If there are tears in the birth canal, with serious bleeding, treat as an open wound by applying direct pressure to the bleeding area with a pad of sterile or clean cloth.

SUPPLIES FOR EMERGENCY CHILDBIRTH

In anticipation of emergency childbirth at home or en route to the hospital, assemble newspapers, plastic bags, or other material to protect bedclothes or car upholstery; clean towels; one or two folded sheets; a set of sterile cord ties or sterilized shoelaces; a new razor blade in protective paper (one-edged); alcohol; scissors; sanitary napkins; a receiving blanket for the baby; a diaper; and safety pins. For a long automobile ride, have the mother wear a nightgown or slip and a robe (no other underclothing) and place a sanitary napkin or clean, folded towel between her thighs if the bag of waters has broken or if blood and mucus are draining from the birth canal. Take along a flashlight, if the trip will be at night; a blanket and pillow; and a container of some sort for the afterbirth.

17

EMERGENCY RESCUE AND TRANSFER

This chapter deals with the movement of victims away from hazardous locations and the use of protective methods to support a victim's body during emergency transfer. Involvement of the first-aider in emergency rescue and transfer is limited to situations in which professional ambulance or rescue personnel and equipment are not or will not be available, to assisting these professionals when they are available, and to removing victims when there is immediate danger to their lives.

If a person is ill or injured to the extent that he will require transport to a medical facility, the first decision to be made by the first-aider is whether it is necessary for the victim to be transferred a short distance before being placed on a litter and in an ambulance. Unless there is immediate danger to the life of the victim from such hazards as those listed below, he should not be transferred until such life-threatening problems as airway obstruction and hemorrhage are cared for, wounds are dressed, and fractures are splinted.

It should be recognized that more harm can be done through improper rescue and transportation than through any other measure associated with emergency assistance. As a rule, rescue from confinement or pinning should be carried out by ambulance or rescue personnel (see chapter 18). Pending their arrival, the first-aider should gain access to the victim, give him emergency care, reassure him, and avoid ill-advised or foolhardy attempts at rescue that might jeopardize the safety of the victim as well as that of the first-aider.

DEFINITION OF EMERGENCY RESCUE

Emergency rescue is a procedure for moving a victim from a dangerous location to a place of safety.

INDICATIONS FOR IMMEDIATE RESCUE

- Fire, danger of fire, or explosion
- Danger of asphyxia due to lack of oxygen or due to gas
- Serious traffic hazards
- Risk of drowning
- Exposure to cold, intense heat, or intense weather conditions
- Possibility of injury due to collapsing walls or building
- Electrical injury or potential injury
- Pinning by machinery

OBJECTIVES

When it is necessary to remove a person from a life-threatening situation, the objectives for the first-aider are—

- To ensure an open airway and to administer artificial respiration if it is needed
- To control severe bleeding
- To check for injuries
- To immobilize injured parts before extrication of the victim
- To arrange for transportation
- To avoid subjecting the victim to any unnecessary disturbance

It is difficult for inexperienced helpers to lift and carry a person gently. They need careful guidance. If there is time, it is wise to rehearse the lifting procedure first, using a practice subject.

IMMEDIATE RESCUE WITHOUT ASSISTANCE

Pulling the Victim

If a person must be pulled or dragged to safety, he should be pulled in the direction of the long axis of his body, preferably from the shoulders (Fig. 199)—not sideways. Every effort must be made to *avoid bending* or twisting his neck or trunk. The danger is less if a board, blanket, or similar object (such as a small rug or a large piece of cardboard) can be placed beneath him, so that he can "ride" the object (Fig. 200). Do not try to lift or carry an injured person before a check for injuries can be made, unless you are sure that there is no major fracture or involvement of his neck or spine.

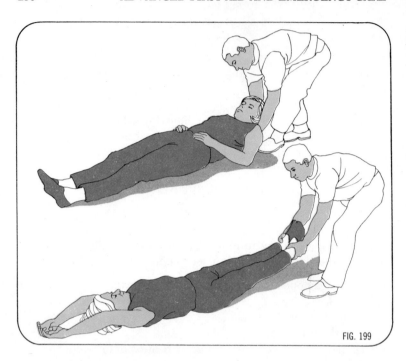

FIG. 199

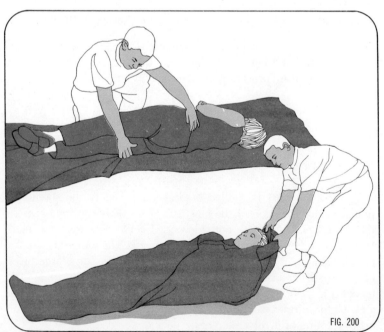

FIG. 200

Lifting the Victim

A lightweight adult or a child who has no serious wounds or skeletal injuries may be carried by one person. Place one hand under his knees and the other under his upper back and armpit for support (Fig. 201).

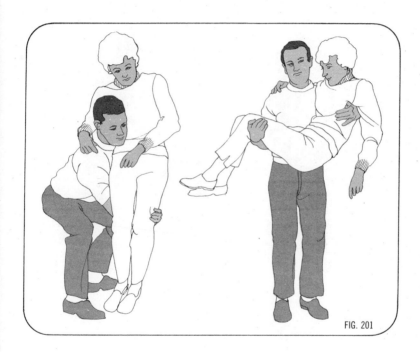

FIG. 201

Supporting the Victim

A person who has no serious wounds or skeletal injuries, who has not had a heart attack, and who is conscious may be assisted to walk to safety. Help him to his feet, place one of his arms around your neck, hold his hand at your chest (or shoulder) level, and place your other arm about his waist for additional support (Fig. 202). An assistant may be used, if available (Fig. 203).

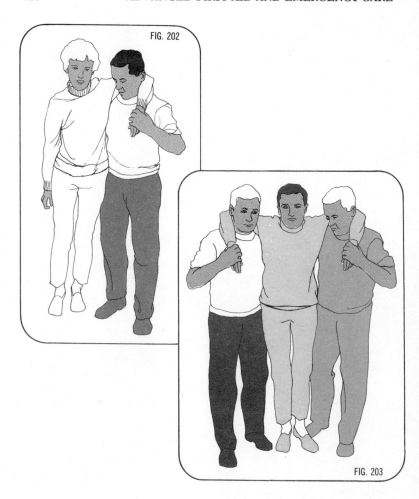

FIG. 202

FIG. 203

IMMEDIATE RESCUE WITH ASSISTANCE

Sometimes, the hazards are so great that it is necessary to move an injured person a short distance without first immobilizing the affected parts. If the victim is to be lifted by several persons, the first-aider should devote himself to the area of greatest injury, protecting it as much as possible. He should prevent bending and twisting of injured parts, such as the limbs, by placing one of his hands just above and on top of the suspected injury and the other just below and under the part, as helpers lift the victim and support the main weight of the limb.

Chair Carry

If a second person is available to assist, but no litter or blanket is available, a convenient technique for carrying a person is to seat him on a strong chair (Figs. 204 and 205). This method is also satisfactory

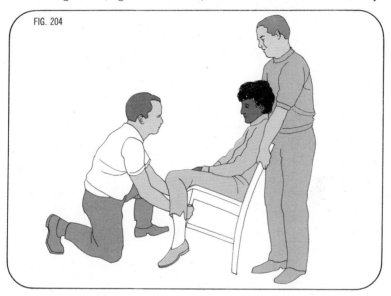

FIG. 204

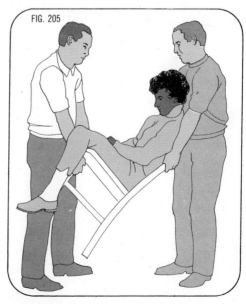

FIG. 205

for going up and down stairs, through narrow corridors, and around corners. This technique is not suitable for persons with neck or back injuries or injuries of the legs.

Fore-and-Aft Carry

The fore-and-aft carry (Figs. 206 and 207) is a two-man technique. It may be used in moving an unconscious person but it is not applicable when there are serious injuries of the trunk or there are fractures.

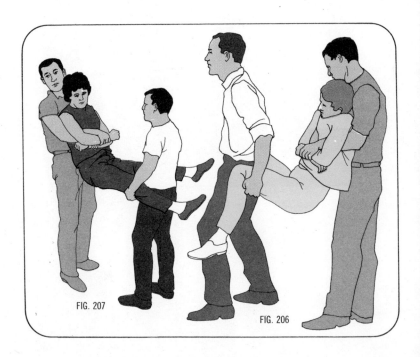

FIG. 207

FIG. 206

Two-Handed and Four-Handed Seats

Another two-man rescue technique is the two-handed seat or swing. If the victim has no serious injuries and is able to cooperate with his rescuers, he may be placed on a two-handed seat, as shown, with his arms about the necks of the first aid workers and his back supported by their free hands (Fig. 208 through 211). Or the four-

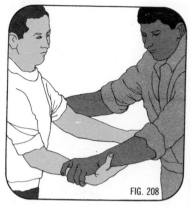

FIG. 208

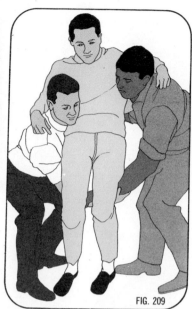

FIG. 209

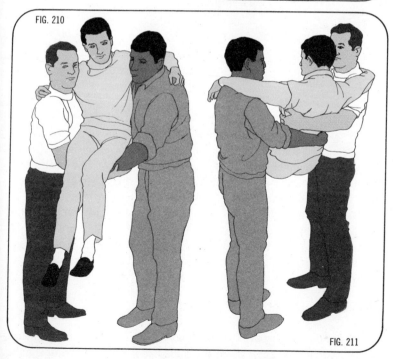

FIG. 210

FIG. 211

handed seat may be used (Fig. 212), in which case better support is provided for seating, but the victim's back is not supported.

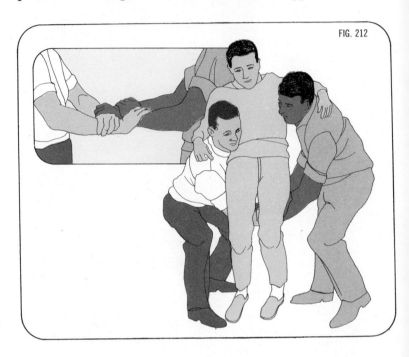

FIG. 212

Blanket Techniques

If transfer is necessary before a litter can be provided, a blanket can be placed under a person for lifting and carrying him a short distance. A blanket should never be used if there is a suspected fracture of the neck or back, unless the hazard is so great that time does not permit procuring a backboard. If the use of a blanket is necessary for a victim with a suspected neck or back fracture, one first aid worker should steady the victim's head, holding traction in a straight line away from the victim's trunk pages 280 and 281, Figs. 242 through 246). If his body is to be turned, it is moved as a unit so that no twisting or side-to-side motion of his neck or back occurs.

Placing Blanket Under Victim From the Side

Allow about two-thirds of the blanket to fall in folds or pleats beside the victim. Then place the folded (not rolled) portion snugly against his body (Fig. 213). Grasp the victim at his hips and shoulders and roll him gently about one-eighth of a turn away from the blanket (Fig. 214). Push the folded part of the blanket as far under the victim as possible and roll him back over the folds and approximately one-eighth of a turn in the opposite direction. Pull the blanket on through (Fig. 215). This procedure places the victim in the middle of the blanket, which can then be rolled from the sides and used to lift him onto a stretcher or to carry him to safety. If

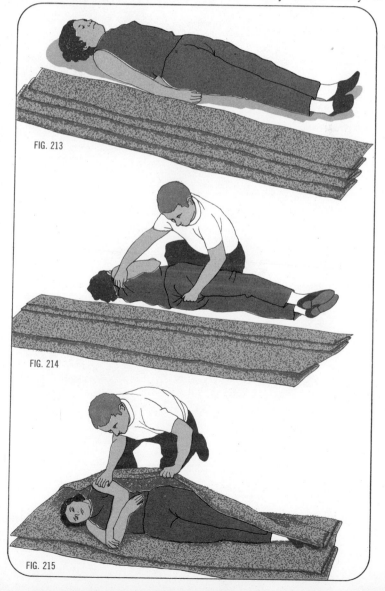

FIG. 213

FIG. 214

FIG. 215

others are available to assist, they should be used (Figs. 216 and 217).

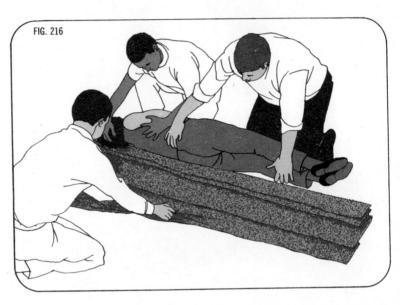

FIG. 216

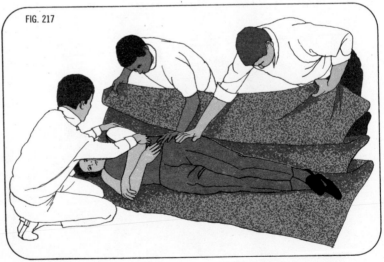

FIG. 217

Blanket Lift

Roll the blanket tightly at the sides until it fits the contours of the victim's body (Fig. 218).

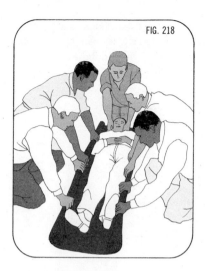

FIG. 218

One person remains at the victim's head, holding slight traction. Two persons at the victim's shoulders grasp the blanket with their top hands at his shoulders and their bottom hands at the upper hip area. The two persons at the lower part of the victim's body grasp the blanket with their top hands at the victim's lower hip area and their lower hands at his legs below his knees (Fig. 219).

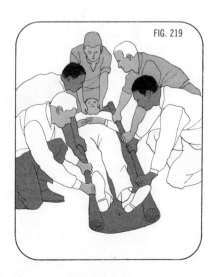

FIG. 219

At a signal, the persons holding the blanket lean back (away from the victim) using their back muscles and body weight (Fig. 220). This action lifts the victim from 6 to 8 inches off the floor or ground so that a litter can be slid underneath. The same procedure is used when a victim is in a prone position.

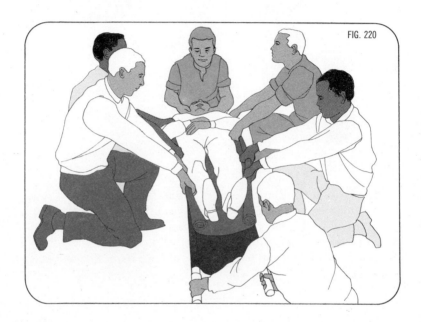

FIG. 220

All parts of the victim's body should be supported—limbs, head, and trunk—and the victim's entire body should be kept immobile and in a straight line. Helpers should lift gradually, following the proper lifting instructions as given, so that they themselves will not suffer back injury. They also should guard against losing their balance. (In all lifts, the leader should give appropriate preparatory signals before the actual signal for action, so that all move as a unit—for example, "Prepare to lift!" and then "Lift!" or "Prepare to stand!" and then "Stand!"

Three-Man Hammock Carry

This technique (Figs. 221 through 224) may be used with the victim on his back (supine) or on his face (prone). In either case, keep his chin up to maintain an open airway.

- Each carrier kneels on his knee that is closer to the victim's feet.
- No. 1 cradles the victim's head and shoulders with his top arm. His other arm is placed under the victim's lower back.
- No. 2—on opposite side from No. 1—slides his top arm under the victim's back *above* No. 1's bottom arm and his other arm just below the victim's buttocks.
- No. 3 slides his top arm under the victim's thighs, above No. 2's bottom arm. His other arm is placed just below the victim's knees (Fig. 221). The hands of No. 1 and No. 2 should be placed about halfway under the victim's body at this stage.
- The command "Prepare to lift!" is followed by the command "Lift!" and the victim is lifted to the carriers' knees and rested there while their hands are slid far enough under the victim to allow rotation of their hands *inward* to secure two interlocking grips (Figs. 222 and 223).
- The command "Prepare to stand!" is followed by the command "Stand!" and all carriers stand erect with the victim (Fig. 224).
- To lower the victim to the ground or onto a litter, reverse the procedure.

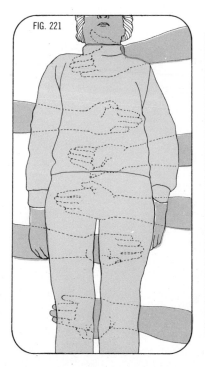

FIG. 221

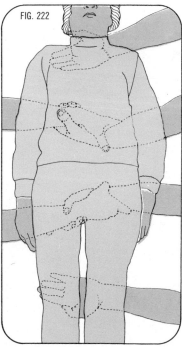

FIG. 222

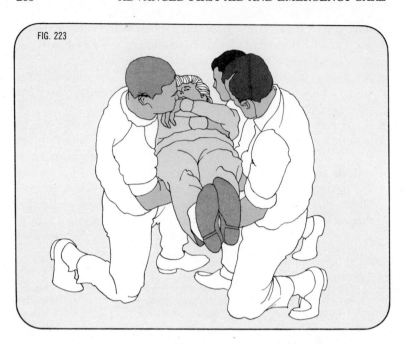

FIG. 223

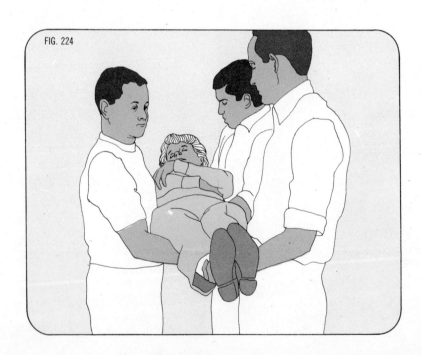

FIG. 224

Three-Man or Four-Man Lift

Three bearers take up positions on one side of the victim and facing him—one at his shoulder, one at his hip, and one at his knee. If one side is injured, the three bearers should be on the victim's uninjured side. (A fourth bearer, if available, takes a position on the opposite side at the victim's hip.)

Each bearer kneels on his knee that is closer to the victim's feet. Then, simultaneously, the bearer at the victim's shoulder puts one arm under the victim's head, neck, and shoulder and the other under the upper part of the victim's back. Each bearer at the victim's hips places one arm under the victim's back and the other under his thighs. The bearer at the victim's knee places one arm under the victim's knees and the other under his ankles (Fig. 225).

The command "Prepare to lift!" is followed by the command "Lift!" and immediately all the bearers lift together and place the victim in line on their knees (Fig. 226).

If there is a fourth bearer, he places a stretcher under the victim and against the toes of the three kneeling bearers. The command "Prepare to lower!" is followed by the command "Lower!" and the victim is gently lowered to the stretcher.

To unload a stretcher, the procedure is reversed. The method described above is also used to place a victim in bed.

When it is necessary to transport a victim in a confined area, he may be carried by three bearers. The victim would then be rolled toward them (Fig. 227).

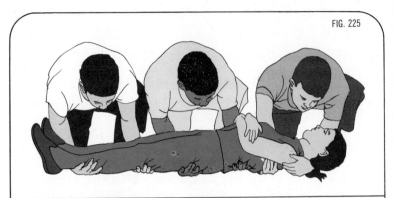

FIG. 225

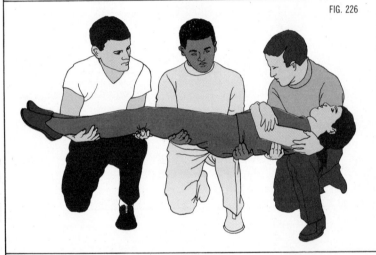

FIG. 226

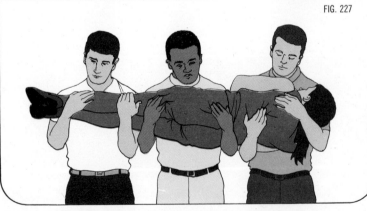

FIG. 227

Six-Man Lift and Carry

There are three bearers on each side of the victim. Each kneels on his knee that is closer to the victim's feet. The bearers' hands, wrists, and forearms are worked gently under the victim until the palms of their hands are about at the midline of the victim's back (or stomach). The hands should be alternated from the two sides. The two hands under the victim's head may have the fingers interlocked to form a cup for his head (Figs. 228 and 229).

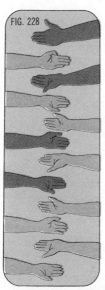

FIG. 228

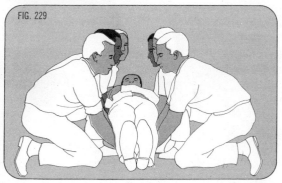

FIG. 229

The command "Prepare to lift!" is followed by the command "Lift!" and the victim is lifted on the bearers' hands and forearms to their knees. Be careful to keep the victim's body in a straight line (Fig. 230). The command "Prepare to stand!" is followed by the command "Stand!" and all bearers stand erect (Fig. 231). To lower the victim to the ground or onto a litter, reverse the procedure. If needed, additional bearers can be placed on both sides of the victim to assist in lifting.

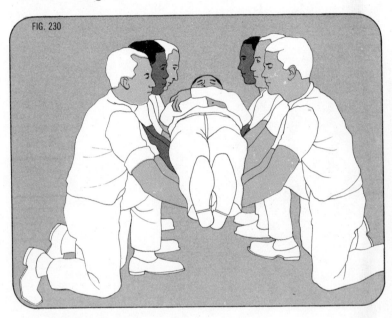

FIG. 230

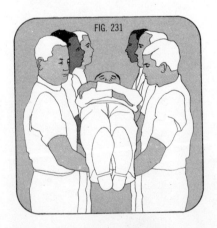

FIG. 231

USE OF STRETCHERS, LITTERS, AND BACKBOARDS

Types

Of the litters shown in Fig. 232, the "army litter" (Figs. 233A through 233D) is most satisfactory for general use. In opening it,

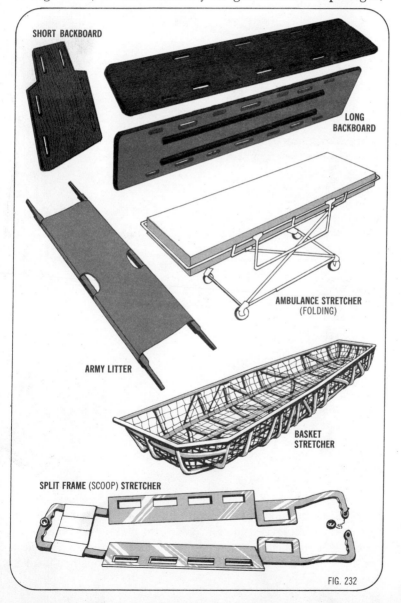

SHORT BACKBOARD

LONG BACKBOARD

AMBULANCE STRETCHER (FOLDING)

ARMY LITTER

BASKET STRETCHER

SPLIT FRAME (SCOOP) STRETCHER

FIG. 232

lock the bracing bars with your foot (Figs. 233B and 233C), if you are wearing shoes, or with the palm of your hand—not by grasping the bar with your hands and fingers. Before using the litter for the victim, test it by lifting someone at least as heavy as the victim.

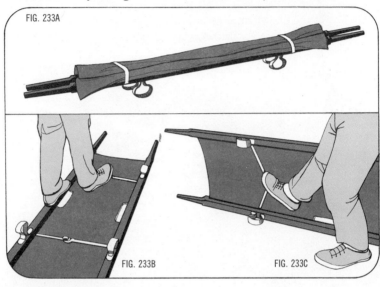

FIG. 233A

FIG. 233B   FIG. 233C

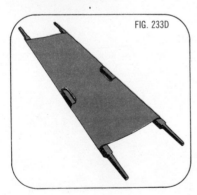

FIG. 233D

Improvised Litter

In an emergency in which ambulance service is delayed or not available, or in remote areas where litters or backboards are not available, an improvised litter may have to be used to transport a person either to shelter or to a source of transportation to a medical facility. A litter may be improvised from clothing, a rug, or a blanket placed over poles (Fig. 234). If available, a lightweight canvas lounge chair, an ironing board, a leaf from a table, or a door may be used. An automobile seat is long enough for a child. Near water, such things as floats, surfboards, and water skis, as well as planks, may be used. Wheeled vehicles can sometimes be used to assist with an emergency litter, and other means of transportation may be used. If an ambulance or rescue vehicle can be brought to the scene, and hazards do not demand transfer, it is better to wait for proper equipment.

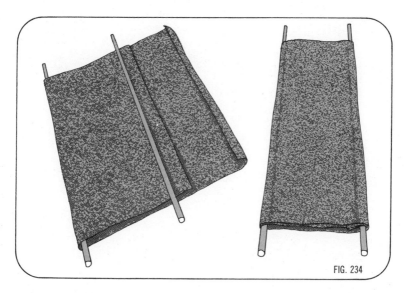

FIG. 234

Carrying Techniques

Care must be taken to secure the injured person or invalid properly, so that he will not roll or slide during transportation. If a neck fracture is suspected, additional padding is necessary to support the victim's head and neck. Use cravat bandages or other improvised ties.

Position of Bearers

It is preferable to have four bearers: one at the victim's head, one at his feet, and one at each side—all facing the direction of intended movement. Each side bearer holds the side of the litter with his hand that is closer to the victim. All assume the proper lifting stance, and at the command "Lift!" all stand erect.

At the command "March!" the bearer at the head of the litter steps off on his right foot, and the bearers at the sides and feet step off on their left feet (Fig. 235). To lower the litter, the bearers reverse the steps used to lift the litter.

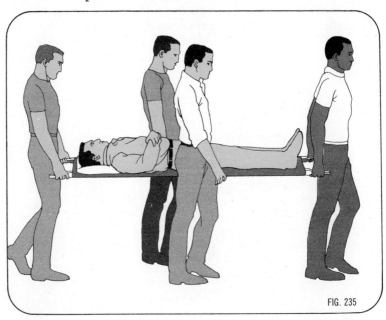

FIG. 235

Use of Backboard

Short and long backboards are essential for immobilization of fractures or suspected fractures of the spine or neck. Backboards are standard equipment on ambulances and rescue vehicles and should be readily available at swimming areas, industrial plants, ski slopes, and other sites where accidental injury is common. Unless emergency rescue justifies removal of such victims from dangerous locations, the first-aider should care for life-threatening conditions while waiting for backboards. The first-aider should be trained to assist ambulance or rescue squad personnel; but if he has to move a victim before professionals arrive, he should use a backboard for immobilization of the victim's spine and neck, for fractures of the pelvis, and as a means of transport in lieu of a blanket, rug, or improvised litter. Once applied, a backboard should be left in place and transported with the victim on a hand-carried litter or wheeled litter and in an ambulance.

If a spinal fracture is not suspected, the long backboard is placed along the victim's side that has sustained the greater injury. The rescuers kneel on the other side of the victim, with the leader at his head and shoulder area, the second rescuer at his trunk and hip area, and the third rescuer at his thigh and leg area. With each rescuer kneeling on his knee that is closer to the victim's feet, the leader extends the victim's near arm over the victim's head and in line with his body and places the victim's far arm alongside and close to the victim's body. The leader, with his arm and hand that are next to the victim's head, reaches under the victim and gently lifts the victim's head from beneath, cradling it on his forearm and hand. Using his free hand, he reaches over the victim again and gets a firm grip on the clothing at the victim's shoulder. The second rescuer reaches over and gets a firm grip on the clothing, somewhat under the victim on the far side, with one hand at midtrunk and the other at the hip area (neither hand at the victim's arm). The third rescuer reaches one hand over and places it somewhat under the victim's midthigh and places his other hand somewhat under the victim's far calf (Fig. 236). At a signal from the leader, all three roll the victim onto his

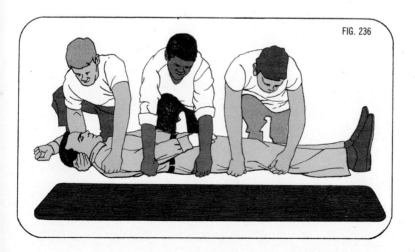

FIG. 236

side toward them, moving him as a unit or solid piece of material. This procedure is referred to as "log rolling" (Fig. 237). When the victim is on his side, the board is placed so that its edge is against his

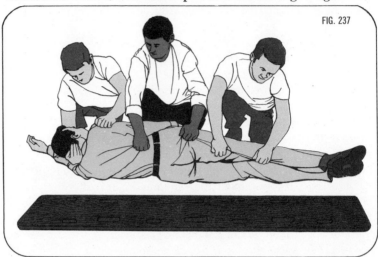

FIG. 237

body. This procedure can be accomplished by another person or by the middle rescuer with whichever hand is convenient (Fig. 238). When the board is in place and the middle rescuer has returned his hand to position, the victim is gently rolled onto the board (Fig.

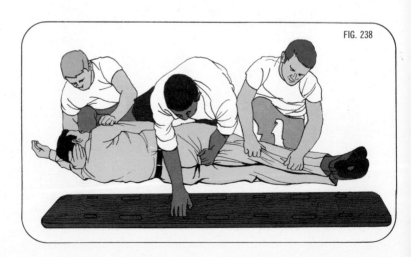

FIG. 238

239). The second man will return the victim's near arm to the
victim's side (Fig. 240). When the victim is secured to the board
with straps, he is ready for transporting (Fig. 241). The board can be

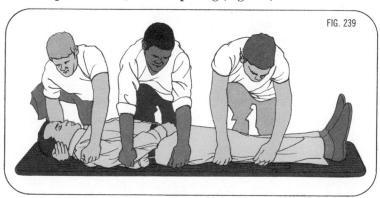

FIG. 239

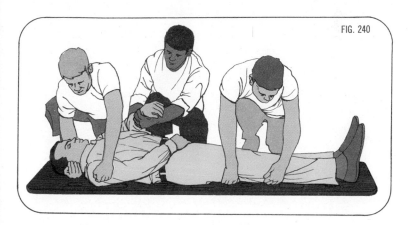

FIG. 240

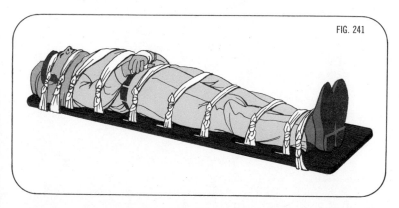

FIG. 241

used for carrying, but carrying the board on a stretcher is easier for any substantial distance.

If an injury to the neck or back is suspected, the victim should be transported flat on his back on a firm frame support. If his body must be turned, it should be turned as a unit, so that no twisting occurs.

If a spinal fracture is suspected, a fourth rescuer is needed to make sure that the victim's head turns with his body as a unit. The fourth rescuer holds the victim's head between his hands and applies slight traction. This action keeps the head in line with the victim's spinal column. This rescuer then becomes the leader and gives the signal for rolling the victim. The rescuer at the victim's shoulder adjusts his hands slightly toward the victim's feet to permit the use of both his hands in the rolling procedure. When the victim is on the board, his head position should be maintained by use of sandbags, triangular bandage ties, or a blanket splint. (Figs. 242 through 246).

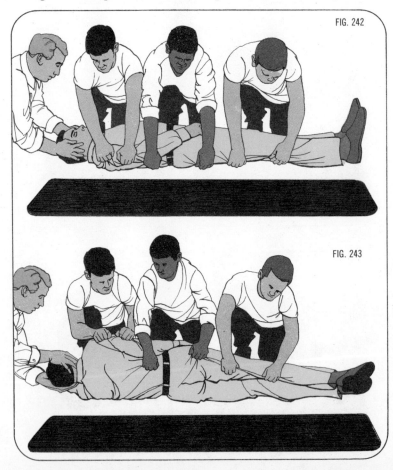

FIG. 242

FIG. 243

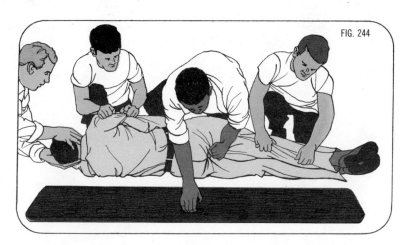

FIG. 244

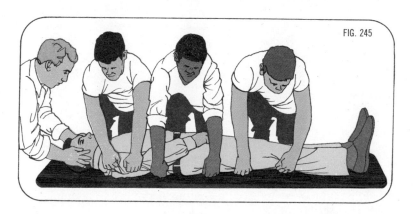

FIG. 245

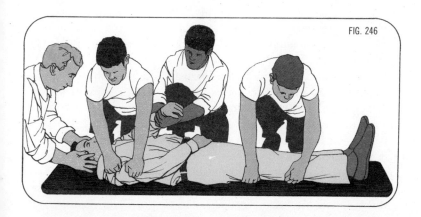

FIG. 246

If the footrest is to be used, it should be placed on the board before the victim is rolled onto it. A measurement should be made so that the footrest will be properly placed (Fig. 247).

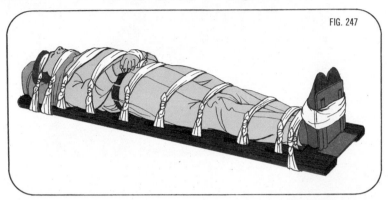

FIG. 247

After a swimming accident in which a fracture of the neck or spine is suspected, the backboard should be floated under the victim, and his head, neck, and body should be immobilized before he is lifted from the water or transferred to a litter (see chapter 6).

Use of Short Backboard

A short backboard is used if the victim is in a sitting position, such as in an automobile seat, if a neck or lower spine fracture (which is common in front-rear automobile accidents) exists or is suspected, or if a situation exists where a long backboard is needed but cannot be applied to the entire length of the body. A short or half backboard should be positioned and secured on the victim before attempts are made to move him.

One first-aider supports the victim's head and body in an upright position, keeping them immobile (Fig. 248), while another places a short board between the victim and the back of the seat, making sure that it is completely inserted to a position lower than the pelvic area (Fig. 249).

Padding is needed between the board and the back of the victim's neck, as well as at the sides of his neck, to provide comfort and to keep the board and neck in position when the victim is moved to a horizontal position. His head is secured to the short board with a cravat bandage across his chin or across his forehead or both, whichever is best, and tied about the notches or through the proper holes in the board. The victim's arms should be placed along his body and secured to the short board with straps—one around his upper chest and one around his waist (Fig. 250).

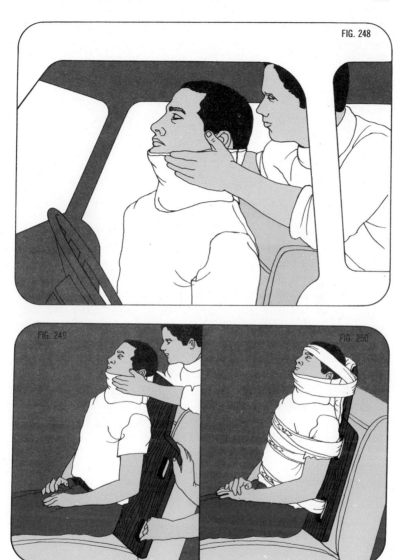

FIG. 248

FIG. 249

FIG. 250

The short backboard is intended for immobilization of the neck and *must not* be used as a handle for lifting a victim. The victim's weight should be borne by the hands of the rescuers, locked under the victim's buttocks. Attempts to lift the victim by using the backboard will result in the victim's sliding down the board with the neck flexed as the neck moves upward behind the occiput (the back part of the skull).

VEHICLE TRANSFER

The first-aider must protect victims of accidental injury or serious illness who require vehicle transfer on a litter against hasty or ill-advised transfer in trucks, station wagons, or any vehicles other than ambulances. On rare occasions, a toboggan or a substitute motor vehicle may be the only means of transport to a site accessible to ambulances. The drive should be at moderate speeds, with gentle stops and starts and with observation of all safety rules. However well-splinted or otherwise immobilized an injured part may be, a fractured or otherwise injured area sustains some harmful effect from the constant swaying and jolting of the vehicle as it rounds turns, slows down, increases speed, or encounters dips and elevations.

Accident victims often benefit from a period of rest before transfer. If the subject is ill, rather than injured, the first-aider customarily has no special preparation responsibilities unless delegated by a physician. Too often, a victim is subject to disturbing and exhausting preparation before transportation is begun.

It is important to remember that people who may have head injuries, fractures of the thigh, leg, arm, or pelvis, or possible back injuries and those with heart attacks or chest or abdominal injuries should not be transported sitting up in automobiles. The injured parts need immobolization; the victim should be recumbent on a comfortable support and should be transported safely.

18

EXTRICATION

In various accident situations, it is impossible for a victim to free himself. He may be confined in an automobile, pinned and held by machinery, or trapped by a cave-in. He may be injured, and there may be danger—known, or unknown but possible—to him or the rescuer. *It is necessary for a first-aider to get to the accident victim whenever possible, to provide life support until persons trained in operating rescue equipment and in taking the proper action in an interruption of utilities (such as electric, gas, and water) can be brought to the scene.*

In some areas of the country, long delays, distance, or the lack of resources to provide essential help may make it necessary for a first-aider to assume the leadership role in extricating victims. He should protect the victim from further injury and maintain life support during the planning and preparation for extrication, as well as during transportation of the victim to the proper emergency medical facilities. To carry out these functions, the first-aider should be familiar with the basic materials and equipment that he may use to obtain access to a victim. For example, in an automobile accident, it may be necessary for him to use such tools as a screwdriver, a crowbar, or a hammer to pry open a door or break a window, or to use a sturdy knife to cut the rubber molding around a window in order to pop it out. In trying to gain entrance to a car or remove its occupants, keep in mind that seats and doors of cars can be removed. Entrance can be through the trunk if the rear seat is removed, and the steering wheel can sometimes be moved out of the way. Caution should be observed to protect the victims from further injury. When cutting and prying windows, the first-aider should wear protective glasses and gloves for his own protection and should cover the victims, if possible.

The first-aider should adapt the principles of first aid to the various situations that require his assistance.

REMOVAL FROM AUTOMOBILE

The following are examples of common rescues of persons from automobile accidents. Methods of releasing the victims can be applied to other accidents that create similar conditions.

Car on Its Side

Spinal injuries are common in accidents in which cars have turned over onto their side. Guard against the impulse to get the car back onto its wheels before the occupants can be removed.

If possible, the first-aider should enter the car to examine an accident victim and to administer emergency first aid. If spinal injury is not suspected, the victim may then be assisted from the car and onto a stretcher. If spinal or neck injury is suspected, a short backboard should be put in place and the victim should be secured to it (see page 283, Figs. 248 through 250). With the board in place, the victim can be raised to an upright sitting position. With two first-aiders in the car and two outside on the side of the car, the long backboard should be placed at the back of the victim as he is raised to a vertical position. Straps should be used to secure him to the board. He can then be hoisted out and laid in a horizontal position on the car. Helpers outside on the ground can take the board and lower it onto a stretcher.

Car Upside Down

Seats and other loose articles should be removed by the person entering the car. The victims *must* be removed before the car is righted. Emergency first aid should be provided by one first-aider while another enters the car to assist in removal. A first-aider working from the outside can also help control movement of the victim's head and neck, if necessary.

If injuries are such that a backboard should be applied, the victim's feet and legs should be tied together with two or three cravat bandages, evenly spaced. The two rescuers can then place the victim on the long board with minimal movement. When he is secured to the board by straps, the board is slid out and placed on a stretcher. Exit should be made through whichever opening is easiest.

Victim Lying on Seat

When a victim is lying on a seat, he is usually on his side with his legs hanging over the seat (Fig. 251A). Having accomplished the necessary first aid, one rescuer holds the victim's head, keeping it immobile and in line with the victim's body (Fig. 251B). Another rescuer attends to the victim's feet and legs, gently moving them into line with the victim's body and keeping them extended (Fig. 251C). If the victim is on the front seat, rescuers enter the rear seat

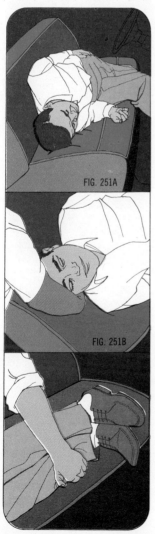

FIG. 251A

FIG. 251B

area and reach over and grasp the clothing of the victim with both hands at evenly spaced intervals from shoulder to thigh. Pulling on his clothing, they gently ease him away from the back of the seat. The backboard is slid into place between the victim and the seat back by other rescuers. Rescuers in the rear ease the victim back against the board (Fig. 251D) and then reach over him and grasp the lower edge of the board, keeping their arms against his body (Fig. 251E). The rescuer at the victim's head reaches over the head and grasps the lower edge of the board, keeping his arm in contact with the victim's forehead to prevent movement (Fig. 251F). The rescuer at the victim's feet reaches over and across the victim's legs to prevent movement (Fig. 251G). The hands of the rescuers at the victim's head and feet who are not involved with control of the victim then grasp the bottom edge of the board. At a signal from the man at the victim's head, all rescuers lift and allow the board to lower gently until flat on the seat. The two rescuers in the rear seat of the car move out to the side of the car and receive the backboard as it is passed out to them.

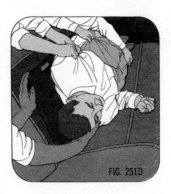

FIG. 251D

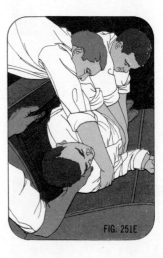

FIG. 251E

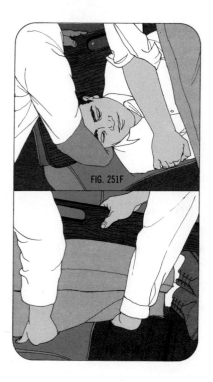

FIG. 251F

Victim in Prone Position

When a victim lying in the prone position has received emergency first aid, he is rolled as a unit onto his side, the board is placed close to and along the full length of his body, and he is rolled onto the board and secured to it.

Victim on Floor in Front

When the victim is on the floor in the front of the car (Fig. 252A), the board is placed on the seat in the desired position. One rescuer

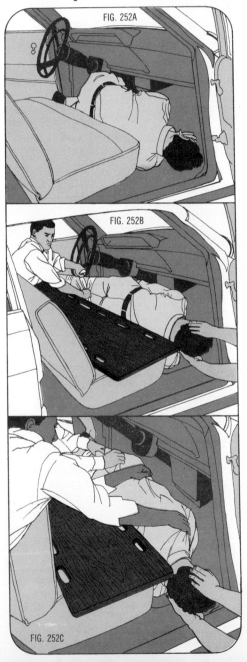

FIG. 252A

FIG. 252B

FIG. 252C

at the victim's head keeps the head and neck in alignment with the body. This action can be best accomplished if the victim's legs are tied together (Fig. 252B). Two rescuers enter the rear of the car; reaching over the back of the seat, they grasp the clothing of the victim at his thigh, hip, waist, and shoulder, making sure the clothing is not torn or loose. They should not grasp the victim's arm (Fig. 252C).

At a signal from the rescuer at the victim's head, all rescuers lift the victim, keeping his body in alignment and against the seat. When his body is high enough, it is gently eased down onto the board (Fig. 252D). The two rescuers in the rear of the car move out of the car to receive the board as it is passed out (Fig. 252E).

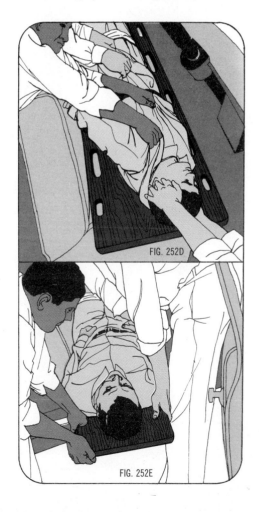

FIG. 252D

FIG. 252E

Victim on Floor in Back

When a victim is on the floor in the rear of the car, the same procedures are used as for a victim on the floor in front, except that the board is placed on the rear seat and two rescuers enter the front seat area and reach over the back of the seat (Figs. 253A through D).

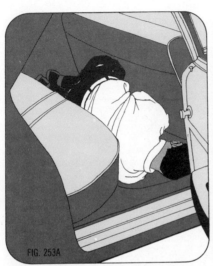
FIG. 253A

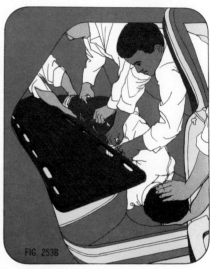
FIG. 253B

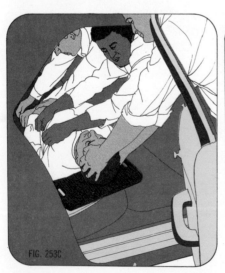
FIG. 253C

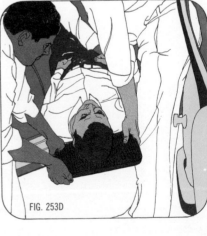
FIG. 253D

If the clothing of the victim does not appear to be strong enough to support him during lifting, place strong cravat bandages around him in appropriate locations. Tie them off and lift the victim by the bandages (Figs. 254A through 254E).

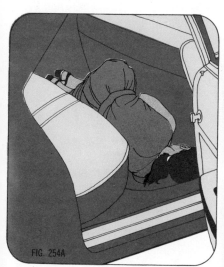

FIG. 254A

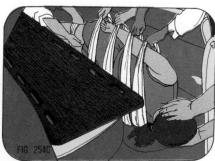

FIG. 254C

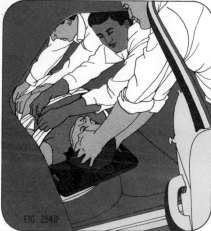

FIG. 254D

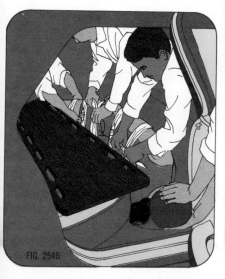

FIG. 254B

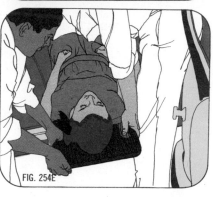

FIG. 254E

Alternate Method for Victim on Floor

There is another way of rescuing a victim on the car floor. One end of the long backboard is placed on the floor in the doorway opening with the other end supported in a level position. The first-aider slides the victim out of the car onto the board by grasping his clothing or using a rope sling around his chest. A helper guides the legs, keeping the traction in line with the long axis of the victim's body, with as little twisting as possible (Fig. 255A). If the board is

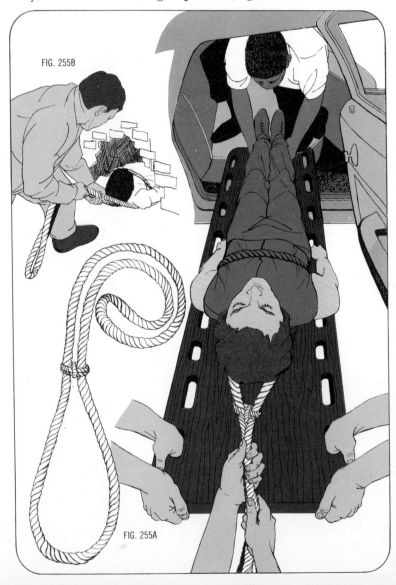

FIG. 255B

FIG. 255A

properly finished, its surface will be highly polished, and even a heavy victim may be easily moved in this manner. A rope sling may also be used to remove a victim from a confined area (Fig. 255B).

NOTE. After any automobile accident in which a spinal fracture is known or suspected, the use of a short backboard is preferred before the victim is moved to a long backboard.

UNUSUAL SITUATIONS

Rescue From Elevation or Excavation

In the rescue of an unconscious or injured person from either an elevation or an excavation, the long backboard can be used if a fracture or some other serious injury requires immobilization. Rescue in the horizontal position, rather than the vertical, is more comfortable for the victim. However, the situation will indicate which position to use.

After emergency first aid has been given, place the victim on the long backboard and prepare him for horizontal hoist (Fig. 256). Secure him to the board by passing the straps through the holes on either side of the board and across him. Thus it is unnecessary to lift the board each time a strap is applied. Secure the victim's head to the board by a cravat bandage across his chin or across his forehead

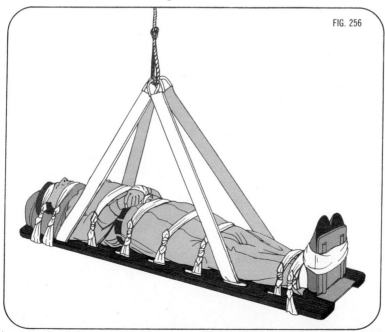

FIG. 256

(or both) tied through the proper holes in the board. Straps should be at the victim's chest area, at his waist, and slightly above his knees. Adjustments may be made, depending on the victim's injuries.

Place a rescue belt through the proper openings of the board. Bring the rings together and secure them over the victim, using the hoisting or lowering line. If a belt is not available, a 3/4-inch line can be used as a suspension loop. The hoisting or lowering line should be a 3/4-inch line. Hoisting or lowering equipment can be a fire department aerial, an industrial crane, or utility "cherry pickers" or "gin poles," erected with either ladders or poles.

The person in charge of the rescue crew should be in charge of the entire procedure. He should not, however, try to tell the operator of mechanical equipment how to operate that equipment. He should indicate what he wants done and how he wants it done. His responsibility is to the injured victim. The use of hand signals by day or flashlight by night is more efficient than shouting instructions. The signals should be predetermined and understood before any action is taken.

When the vertical hoist (Fig. 257) is to be used, the straps secur-

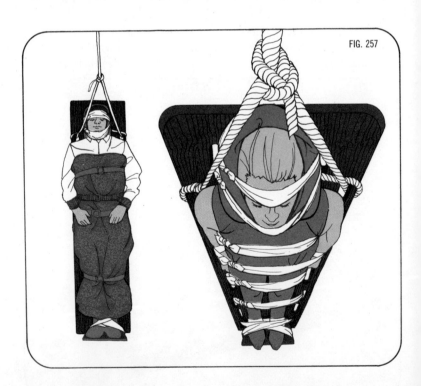

FIG. 257

ing the victim's body to the board must be placed through the appropriate openings in the board and over the victim's body. The top strap should be placed under the victim's armpits and over his chest. Locations for the other two straps are as described for the horizontal hoist. The footrest must be used and the victim's feet secured to it with a cravat bandage.

As a rule, long boards do not have a footrest; but even if they do, leg fractures would make it undesirable for the victim's weight to be supported against the footrest. The victim should be secured to the board by the long straps passing about his thighs high in his groin and across his body over the opposite shoulder and being secured to holes in the board. Additional straps may be placed about his body at the chest level and knees. The victim's head is secured by a cravat bandage over his chin or forehead (or both), which is tied through the appropriate holes in the board. The hoisting line should be laced through openings at the upper third of the board, with the securing knot to the front of the board. This procedure keeps the board in a vertical position.

In either the horizontal or vertical rescue, two guidelines should be used to prevent swinging and twisting of the board while it is being raised or lowered.

Cave-Ins

Extreme caution must be exercised at a cave-in accident. Because the location of the victims may not be readily apparent, additional injury may be caused through the loosening of additional material. The possibility of causing such injury must be avoided. Onlookers must be kept well away from the immediate area.

The first-aider should evaluate the situation and determine what must be done. He should distribute his weight over as wide an area as possible, even to lying down as he nears the edge of the excavation. The probable location of the victim must be determined, and then efforts must be directed to uncovering his face and chest. The uncovering is best done with long-handled shovels that permit the rescuers to stand a little away from the victim.

When the victim's head and face are free, artificial respiration should be started, if it is necessary. Supportive care with oxygen should be administered if oxygen and a person trained to use it are available. Efforts to uncover the victim's chest and the remainder of his body must continue.

Once the victim is completely free, and if his injuries require immobilization, he should be placed on a backboard and brought out of the excavation. The excavation may not be deep enough to require mechanical equipment to do the hoisting; but, in any event, the victim should be properly secured to the board before he is brought out. He can then be placed on a stretcher and transported to the nearest medical facility.

Accidents Involving Machinery

People are sometimes accidentally pinned in or under machinery. These accidents may entail severe lacerations and avulsions, multiple fractures, or severe burns. There may be severe traumatic shock. Emergency first aid should be given promptly. If release will not be possible for a long period, it is advisable to get a physician to the scene to administer medical care.

The machinery should be stopped and the power cut off. A person familiar with the operation of the machine would probably know how to release the victim. The machine may have an automatic releasing device. If not, it can be dismantled. A section of the machine may have to be removed, with the victim still pinned, and transported to the hospital, where the victim may have to undergo surgery. On-the-spot surgery may be the only way to release him; this surgery is to be decided upon and performed by a physician.

During the entire procedure, one first-aider attends the victim, controlling hemorrhage, treating for shock, reassuring, keeping the victim's airway open if he becomes unconscious, and doing whatever else is needed to make the victim as comfortable as possible.

Structural Collapse

In the structural collapse type of accident, there are several possible situations:

* The victim may simply be confined.
* The atmosphere may be oxygen-deficient, explosive, or toxic.
* The victim may be pinned.
* The victim may be injured.
* Communication with the victim may not be possible.

The safety of the first-aiders must be an important consideration in the rescue of a victim from a structural collapse. The exact or probable location of the victim should be established, and then the procedures for rescue can be worked out.

If the victim can be reached, emergency first aid should be given as necessary and plans made for proper removal. In the event of other than very minor fractures, the use of a backboard is in order. Using the backboard will make moving more comfortable for the victim and reduce the risk of additional injury.

Toxic or Oxygen-Deficient Atmosphere

First-aiders should not attempt rescues from toxic or oxygen-deficient atmosphere unless the area has been thoroughly ventilated or they have proper equipment for respiratory protection. Self-contained air or oxygen equipment is recommended, because rescuers cannot be sure whether the atmosphere has enough oxygen to sustain life.

Both high and low ventilation are required, because poisonous gases may be either heavier or lighter than air. The use of fans (either blower or suction) will aid in ventilation, removing gases and vapors from the area. Electric fans should not be used in an area where flammable gases may be present. It is advisable to have a lifeline attached to any rescuer entering a dangerous atmosphere. This line should lead to the outside and should be attended by another person. Predetermined signals should be used at short intervals for ascertaining the status of a rescuer. Rescues of this kind will have to be made at the risk of possible additional injury, but additional injury can be minimized by moving the victim on the long axis of his body (lengthwise).

Impaled Victims

Accidents in which victims become impaled most often involve children at play. The objects on which they become impaled include fence spikes, tree branches, and furniture, toys, bicycles, automobiles, and construction equipment with pointed projections.

If the victim has not been removed from the impaling object when the first-aider arrives, the first action should be to relieve the strain on the victim's body. First aid should be given for airway obstruction or bleeding.

If at all possible, the part of the object upon which the person is impaled should be removed from the rest of the object. This removal is done by dismantling, cutting with a hacksaw, or in whatever other way is most simple. The victim should be transported in the most comfortable manner possible while the object remains in his body, with the object padded and immobilized with massive dressings (see pages 39 and 40) and secured to minimize movement. *The first-aider will cause additional injury if he removes the object from the victim, or the victim from the object.*

Electrical Emergencies

Whatever the cause of an electrical emergency—electric wires in the home, high-tension wires on the street, a bolt of lightning or anything else—electric shock can cause an emergency if it paralyzes the breathing center in the victim's brain or produces unconsciousness. Upon rescue, give the victim artificial respiration and treat him for shock. Cardiopulmonary resuscitation may be necessary but it should be applied only by specially trained persons. After successful resuscitation, keep the victim absolutely still until he can be moved to a hospital for further observation and treatment of electrical burns that might have occurred.

In the Home

Electrocution from low-voltage current is common in the home. The danger in the home is often underestimated, especially the danger to the rescuer if he touches the same equipment or the injured person. The rescuer should disconnect the attachment plug from its socket or throw the main house electric switch, if possible.

Fallen Wire on Vehicle

The best action in a situation involving a fallen wire on a vehicle is to calm the occupants and get them to remain inside the vehicle until professional rescue workers arrive. It is rare that fire or other circumstances warrant emergency rescue. If so, however, the first-aider should calm the occupants and tell them that he will instruct them on how to get out and that they should make no moves other than as directed. Instruct *the person in the front seat* to do as follows:

• Open the door on the passenger side as wide as possible, being careful that it does not touch the ground.
• Slide the front seat as far to the rear as it will go.
• Turn to face the door, keeping your feet in the vehicle.
• Move to the edge of the seat.

- Fold your arms across your chest and hold the upper part of each arm with the opposite hand.
- Make sure that your head is out from under the roof.
- Get ready to jump; and when you are ready, jump with both feet at the same time, as far out as possible.
- Walk quickly away.

Repeat this procedure with each person, having each person climb out in turn.

INDEX

definition, 151
signs and symptoms and first aid, 152
Heel bone (calcaneus) fractures, 188–89
Hemorrhages (hemorrhaging), 232–33
  aorta, 28
  brain injury, 50
  control in fractures, 158, 161, 164, 169
  description, signs, and symptoms, 232–33
  dressings and bandages, 202–24
  face and jaw injuries, 51
  first aid, 233
  head injuries, 49, 50
  internal injuries, 27, 43, 232–33
  and pregnancy, 247
  and shock, 59, 60, 61
  stopping, 30–38
    direct pressure, 30–33
    elevation, 30, 33
    tourniquet, 30, 36–38
  See also Bleeding, severe
Hemorrhoids ("piles"), 241
  bleeding, 232
  first aid, 241
  rectal pain, 241
Hernia, and abdominal pain, 239–40
  strangulated, 239
Heroin, 128
  abuse, 131
Hiccups, 244
Hip and thigh (femur) fractures, 169, 170, 182–84
  bandages, 205
  reference illustration, 183
  tractions splints for, 194–201
Hip wounds, bandages for, 213
Hornet (hornet stings), 108–9
Household (home environment) accidents
  drowning, 83
  electricity, 300
  falls and fractures, 157
  fires and burns, 134, 143
  poisoning, 95–96, 97
  swallowed objects, 66
Household chemicals, and poisoning, 95–96, 97
  See also specific kinds
Hyperglycemia, 230
Hyperventilation, as cause of drowning, 85
Hypoglycemia, 231–32

Ice skating, and water accidents, 83, 94
  rescue, 94
Identification
  medical, 22, 23
  of victim, 22, 23
Illnesses, sudden. See Sudden illness; specific emergencies, kinds
Immobilization
  in closed fractures, 45
  in dislocations, 190
  emergency rescue and transfer and, 276–84
  in extrication (rescues), 287, 295, 298, 300
  in fractures, 162, 169, 194
  impaled objects and, 39, 300

in infected wounds, 41
  neck vertebrae fractures, 166–69
  in snakebites, 115
Impaled objects (impaled victims), 39
  extrication of, 299–300
Improvised fixed-traction splint, 199–201
Incisions (cuts), 26
  causes, 26
  first aid, 28
Infection, wounds and, 24, 25, 27, 28, 38–40ff.
  bites and, 41–43
  cleansing wounds, 38
  definition, 40
  dressing the wound, 40
  fractures and, 156, 158
  interim emergency care, 41
  pain associated with, 242
  prevention of, 38–40
  rabies, 41, 42–43
  removing foreign bodies, 38–39
  symptoms, 40
  tetanus (lockjaw), 40, 42
Ingested poisons, 95, 96–100
  antidotes, 99
  first aid, 98–100
  food poisoning, 96, 237–38
  inducing vomiting, when and when not to, 98, 99, 100
  poisonous shellfish, 104–5
  signs and symptoms, 96–98
Inhalants, 120, 127–28
  effects, 127
  first aid, 128
  See also Inhalation
Inhalation
  and burns, 135
  inhaled poisons, 100–2
    first aid, 101–2
    sources, 101–2
  superheated air and poisonous gases, 135
  See also Inhalants
Injuries
  accidental. See Accidents (accidental injury); specific kinds
  bone and joint. See Bone and joint injuries
  causes (general), 19
  extrication (rescues) and, 254–84, 285–301
    See also Extrication of victim(s) from accident situations; Rescue, emergency (and transfer)
  first aid, general directions, 20–23
  first aid training, 18, 21–23
  prevention, general, 20
  respiratory emergencies and, 65
  safety awareness and, 19–20
  specific injuries. See Injuries, specific; specific kinds
  urgent care, general, 21
  wounds, 24–45
    See also Wounds
Injuries, specific, 46–58
  abdomen, 56
  back, 56–57